NOURISHING BABY FOOD COOKBOOK

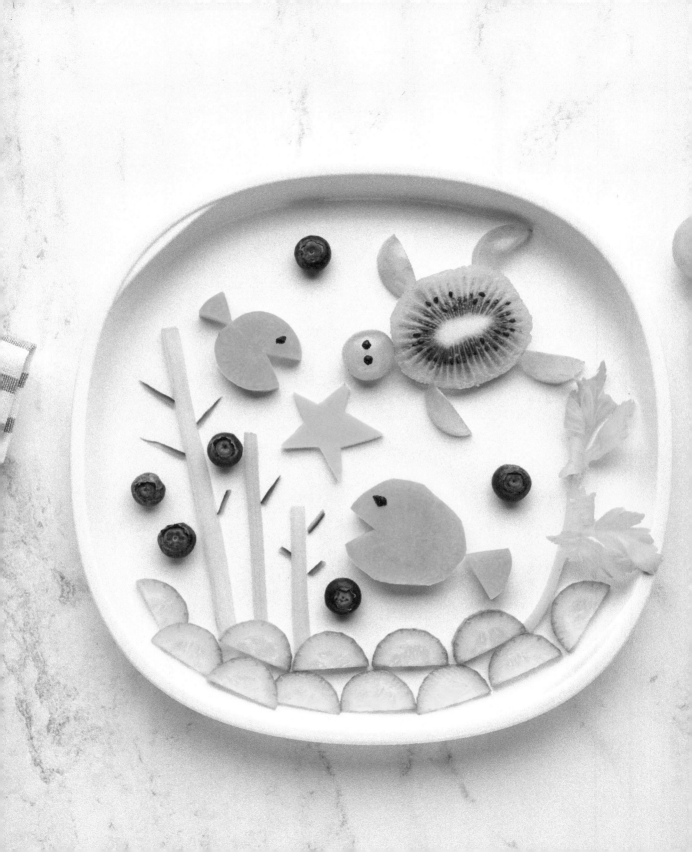

NOURISHING BABY FOOD COOKBOOK

Recipes and Stage-by-Stage
Advice to Achieve Super
Nutrition for Babies

Yaffi Lvova, RDN

Photography by Darren Muir

ROCKRIDGE
PRESS

For general information on our other products and services or to obtain technical support, please contact our Customer Care Department within the United States at (866) 744-2665, or outside the United States at (510) 253-0500.

Rockridge Press publishes its books in a variety of electronic and print formats. Some content that appears in print may not be available in electronic books, and vice versa.

TRADEMARKS: Rockridge Press and the Rockridge Press logo are trademarks or registered trademarks of Callisto Media Inc. and/or its affiliates, in the United States and other countries, and may not be used without written permission. All other trademarks are the property of their respective owners. Rockridge Press is not associated with any product or vendor mentioned in this book.

Interior and Cover Designer: Erik Jacobsen
Art Producer: Sara Feinstein
Editor: Laura Apperson
Production Editor: Sigi Nacson
Production Manager: Jose Olivera
Photography © 2021 Darren Muir. Food styling by Yolanda Muir.

ISBN: Print 978-1-64876-618-3
eBook 978-1-64876-117-1

R0

THIS IS DEDICATED TO THE NEW PARENT.
FEED JOYFULLY.

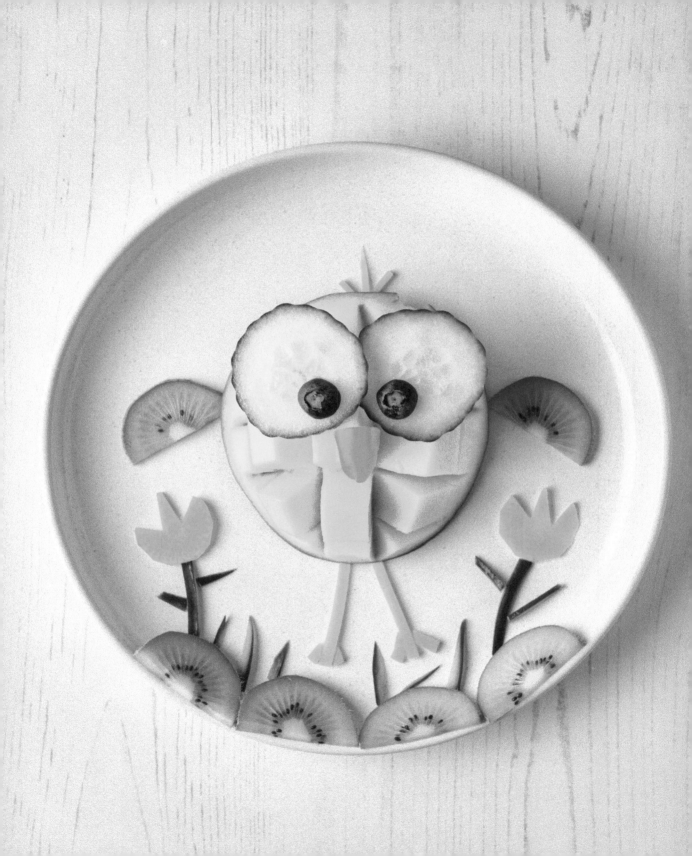

CONTENTS

Introduction xi

1

THE KEYS TO IDEAL NUTRITION 1

2

APPROXIMATELY 6 MONTHS
SINGLE-INGREDIENT PUREES 15

3

6 TO 8 MONTHS
COMBINATION PUREES 43

4

9 TO 12 MONTHS
SMOOTHIES AND SOFT FINGER FOODS 71

5

12 TO 18 MONTHS
TODDLER MEALS 99

6

18 MONTHS AND UP
FAMILY MEALS 125

IF THE HOME IS A BODY,
THE TABLE IS THE HEART,
THE BEATING CENTER,
THE SUSTAINER OF LIFE
AND HEALTH.

—SHAUNA NIEQUIST

INTRODUCTION

HI THERE! I'm Yaffi Lvova, a Registered Dietitian Nutritionist (RDN) focused on increasing laughter at the kitchen table. Parenthood is full of choices, and sometimes it can feel as though each choice is a landmine, resulting in confusion, guilt, and shame.

My goal for this book is to help you feel confident about the choices you make for your child's nutrition so you can cultivate in that child a love for food. Food enjoyment supports nutritional adequacy, as it uses a child's natural curiosity to stimulate exploration of a variety of flavors and textures. At the same time, food is a wonderful springboard for conversations about culture, tradition, and identity. Food can be used to teach math, science, and early literacy. And it all starts with that first bite.

I wasn't always on top of this research. When I gave birth to my twins, seven years ago as of this writing, I had no clue. Sure, I learned in school that babies start eating around 6 months, and was familiar with the basics of Ellyn Satter's Division of Responsibility, but I soon discovered that the reality of becoming a parent and being responsible for feeding babies was not within my comfort zone. I was lost. I was nervous. And I felt crushed by the weight of so many decisions.

I'm thankful to be part of a tight-knit community where I learned how to cross the bridge from textbook to reality. The strong women around me showed me how to care for my babies while caring for myself. And they taught me how to feed my kids, too. After seeing how successful their methods were, I went back to the books and found a wealth of evidence-based research that supports the positive feeding dynamic they were advocating. I discovered baby-led weaning and responsive feeding techniques. Of course, the women who ultimately taught me how to go about doing all this didn't call it by these fancy academic terms. They just called it "dinnertime."

In this book, I explain the common food-introduction timing and methods, debunking any of the crazy feeding mysteries and rumors that may be fueling some food-related anxieties. This science-backed research will serve to allow you to sit back, relax, and enjoy food with your child, reveling in the joy of the impromptu avocado facial or beet-stain kisses. Let's lay the anxiety to rest and get back to "dinnertime."

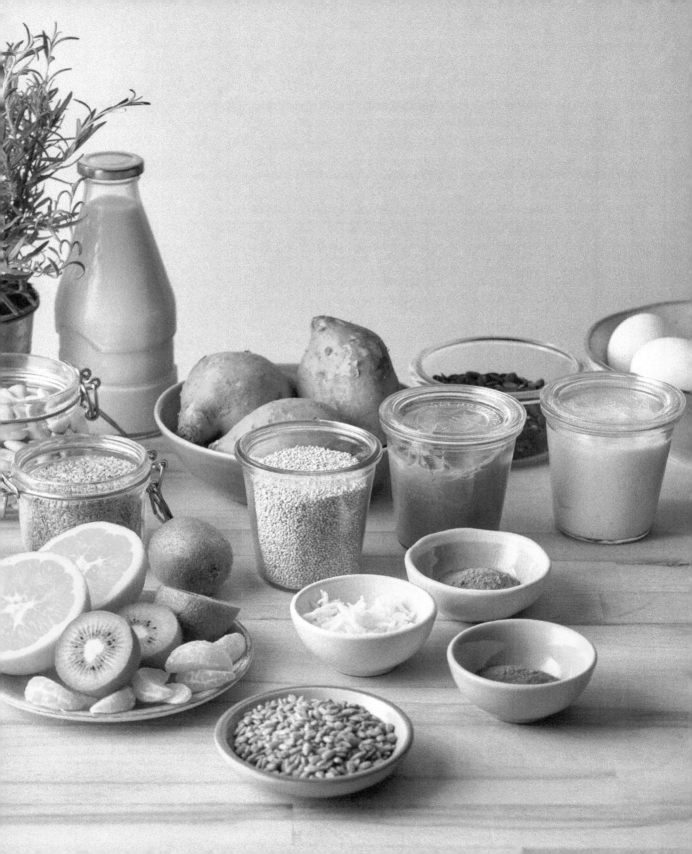

1

THE KEYS TO
IDEAL NUTRITION

Sharing fun experiences with your little one is the best part of parenting. Watching their face light up as they experience something you've enjoyed can take you right back to your own childhood, allowing you to share in the wonder and delight of simple food enjoyment.

SOLID FOOD: AT THE RIGHT TIME

Before jumping in headfirst (or fist-first), remember that there are risks associated with introducing food too early or waiting too long. Luckily, it's pretty easy to tell when your baby is ready.

HOW TO KNOW BABY IS READY

Babies who are ready for solid foods display very specific signs. This happens at around 6 months, but generally not earlier. These signs indicate developmental readiness, showing that your baby can safely eat and absorb food. When your baby is ready for food, they will:

1. Show interest in food.

2. Physically move food from the front of the mouth to the back without pushing it out.

3. Attempt chewing or gumming food.

4. Work toward their pincer grasp, a skill that won't be perfected until around 9 months.

5. Sit up without assistance.

Introducing solids too early has been associated with increased risk for choking, as the very young baby can't move their neck to manage the spit-up of partially digested foods. It has also been associated with increased risk for food allergies, obesity, inadequate growth and development, and other health concerns. However, waiting too long can delay important flavor and texture exposure while postponing essential development of the oral muscles, which will be important for eating and language acquisition.

The two main food-introduction philosophies right now are purees and baby-led feeding (or baby-led weaning). While both methods are safe, consider your comfort level as a parent or caregiver. Food should be presented with joy, not anxiety. If you feel more confident with purees or with baby-led feeding, honor that feeling and feed your child joyfully.

In this book, I introduce you to responsive feeding, a method that works with either purees or baby-led feeding. With this philosophy, you can allow baby to lead the way, whether you're spoon-feeding, providing whole foods, or doing a combination (my personal favorite method). This book starts with purees and introduces more complex foods closer to 12 months, but if you would like to pursue a combination of purees and baby-led feeding, check out my book *Stage-by-Stage Baby Food Cookbook*.

Food as Medicine

Presenting a variety of foods in both color and texture is an easy way to set your baby up for success, as it contributes to overall good health. The many nutrients these various foods provide help to ward off sickness and ensure regular dirty diapers. But it's also okay not to be perfect. In fact, following rules rigidly often leads to anxiety. And anxiety is not the path to good health. There is no single, perfect path to good health but, rather, there are many choices and many ways to present nutritious food. Take this time to enjoy different food experiences with your baby, and as your baby grows, they will be able to appreciate both the crunch of a crisp cucumber slice and the joy of a cup of hot chocolate on a rainy day. Comprehensive health includes being able to relish a variety of delicious food experiences.

THE BEST FOOD FOR BABY

In this book, you'll find stage-specific information to guide you as your baby grows and develops. Here, I explain the pillars of ideal nutrition for baby—concepts you can call on when creating your shopping lists or meal plans. These concepts are meant to relieve any tension that may accompany your meal planning. You are not expected to hit all the nutritional points in any single meal; instead, nutrition needs are met over the course of a few days. After all, it's a marathon, not a sprint!

ESSENTIAL NUTRIENTS

Until baby is about 12 months old, breast milk or formula is the primary source of nutrition. Until your baby is 6 months old, breast milk or formula provides the only required nutrition. At around 6 months, though, when baby shows readiness signs for solids, the iron that was stored in baby's liver from before birth begins to run out. Iron and zinc are nutrients that need to be obtained from solid foods starting at the 6-month stage. Vitamin D is also a concern now, and owing to its lack of availability in many food sources, the National Institutes of Health recommends daily supplementation of 400 IU of vitamin D from birth to 12 months and 600 IU from 1 year to 70 years.

COLORFUL FRUITS AND VEGGIES

Variety is the spice of life! The vibrant and varying colors in fruits and vegetables indicate their unique nutritional offerings. The colors of green, red, blue, purple, orange, and white each indicate a different set of nutrients with their unique health benefits. By offering your baby the full rainbow, you not only provide all that delicious nutrition but also provide a sensory experience that is satisfying on all levels.

A VARIETY OF PROTEINS

At this stage, there is no need to become stressed about the actual amount of protein your baby eats. Protein needs are often exaggerated. For example, a 6-month-old at the 50th percentile of weight requires only about 8.4 grams of protein per day, which is mainly met with breast milk or formula.

However, providing a variety of protein sources does serve to broaden exposure and develop oral muscle. Consider that many high-quality protein sources are commonly overlooked. You can feel confident offering your baby tofu, beans, dairy, nuts and seeds (with certain safety precautions against choking), eggs, and meat as first foods.

Remember that whatever foods you offer right now soon become familiar. This is important as baby grows, since they may experience food neophobia closer to 12 to 18 months. Food neophobia is a fear of new foods. This is a phase that many babies experience around the time they take their first steps (see page 104).

FIBER-RICH WHOLE GRAINS

Whole grains, which are perfectly digested and absorbed at the 6-month mark, provide a wealth of nutrition and can be among the first foods introduced. Including whole grains in the diet sets baby up for reduced risk of developing diabetes, heart disease, and high blood pressure. Fiber, vitamins, minerals, protein, antioxidants, and various plant compounds such as polyphenols, stanols, and sterols all contribute to greater health in the young and old alike. Some super options for whole grains include oatmeal, millet, quinoa, rice, bulghur, buckwheat, barley, and freekeh. These grains can be served as a porridge or used in baked goods.

HEALTHY FATS AND OILS

Research on the Mediterranean style of eating has time and again proven that fat, previously demonized, is essential for growing brains, absorbing certain vitamins and minerals, and manufacturing hormones. Fat also provides a protective effect for multiple organs, helping ward off cardiovascular disease and diabetes. Healthy fats and oils are an important source of energy and can be included in baby's nutrition in many ways, such as including nuts and seeds in your recipes, cooking with a variety of oils, enjoying avocado, and choosing full-fat dairy products until at least age 2.

Allergies, Intolerances, and Sensitivities

Food allergies are immune-system responses to food proteins, while food intolerances and sensitivities are nonimmune reactions. Actual incidence of allergies is less common than you may think. Food allergies that are passed from one generation to the next aren't a specific food allergy; rather, they represent an increased risk that the child will react to a particular food.

The most common *allergens*, causing 90 percent of all allergic reactions, are called The Big 8:

- Cow's milk
- Soy products
- Eggs
- Wheat
- Peanuts
- Tree nuts (Note: Coconut is not included in this allergen, as most people allergic to tree nuts can safely eat coconut.)
- Shellfish
- Fish

Current research shows that introducing these foods early on can minimize the risk of a reaction to them later. If there's a significant history of food allergies in the immediate family, introduce low-allergenic foods two to three days apart and higher allergenic foods (The Big 8) one week apart, with nothing new introduced during that same week. Immediately address reactions to food, such as coughing, wheezing, or swollen lips, keeping in mind that the severity of a reaction can grow more intense from one exposure to the next.

Food *intolerances*, which cannot be tested with a standard allergy test, include lactose and gluten. Symptoms of food intolerance may include gas, constipation, diarrhea, nausea, headaches, eczema, rash around the mouth or in the diaper area, hives, or welts. The child's reactions can indicate either a food allergy, an intolerance, or a sensitivity, and can be mild or more serious. Discuss suspected food reactions with your pediatric dietitian.

If introducing allergenic foods causes you anxiety, choose to time these introductions to coincide with a wellness check at the pediatrician's office. For example, smear your baby's gums with a tiny bit of peanut butter before getting out of the car for the well-check. Should there be cause for concern, the child is already in a safe place.

FLAVORFUL HERBS AND SPICES

Herbs and spices play an important role in the flavor and color of food, but there is significant evidence that they also provide antimicrobial, antioxidant, and anti-tumorigenic properties. Cinnamon, turmeric, and garlic are not only amazing flavor boosters but are also proven to help manage blood sugar, decrease inflammation, and protect the heart and other organs from damage that can lead to disease. Around the world, parents are feeding their babies flavorful and seasoned foods to encourage food enjoyment, impart culture, and encourage good health. Consider adding fresh or dried seasonings to your baby's food, remembering that your little one was already exposed to these flavors in the womb as they tasted the amniotic fluid that sustained them before birth.

NUTRITIOUS BABY FOOD

Providing your baby with the best possible nutrition can be a food adventure for you, too. Join your child in this exploratory journey and you just might find new flavors that make you smile right along with that gummy grinner in front of you.

HOMEMADE VS. STORE-BOUGHT

Offering homemade baby food puts you in the driver's seat. You can select fresh, in-season, and even local produce to truly maximize your baby's flavor exposure and nutrition. This also gives you the opportunity to have your baby with you in the kitchen. While roasting broccoli, lead your little one to experience the feel of the smooth stalk and the flowery top. This is exposure to a new food in a way that baby food from a jar can't match. Also, packaged pureed food is often pricier than homemade food. And if you look carefully, you'll notice that there are some foods that just aren't ever represented in those jars—avocado and melon, for example. There is another important ingredient missing in store-bought food: culture. When feeding your baby homemade food, you can give your little one a taste of what characterizes your family heritage.

But store-bought food isn't all bad. With prepackaged food comes convenience, easy storage, and time savings. Not only is it less time-consuming to purchase baby food, but it also stores easier and lasts longer than homemade versions. If you end up selecting store-bought food sometimes, that's fine! Here are some guidelines to select the best baby foods possible:

CHOOSE FOOD THAT INCLUDES PROTEIN AND FAT. Beans and yogurt are increasingly common additions to baby food, rounding out their nutritional offerings.

AVOID SNEAKY SWEETENERS. No baby food will have "added sugar," but you'll see "evaporated orange juice" in the ingredient list. Babies don't need added sweets; the fruits and veggies in the jar are sweet enough for their sensitive palates.

SHOP THE SALES. All baby food has to meet specific safety standards, so you can feel comfortable buying different brands and different flavors.

WHOLE FOODS FOR BABY

What exactly is meant by "whole foods"? It's the idea of using the entire food item rather than just part of it, keeping it closest to its natural, complete state. These are foods that are either unprocessed or minimally processed. For example, whole wheat flour uses the entire wheat grain, including the outer husk, unlike all-purpose flour, which is processed to remove the husk. If you use whole grains, babies and adults alike can reap the benefits that come with increased fiber and nutrients. By focusing on the intake of whole foods, then, you can make your meals more flavorful and satisfying by using whole grains and fresh fruits and vegetables.

Lemon, garlic, rosemary, and oregano are natural preservatives as well as flavorings, and including them in your homemade baby food can ensure it lasts a bit longer.

HOW TO MAKE HOMEMADE PUREES

Making homemade baby food is easy, is economical, and can help set baby up for lifelong food enjoyment. All you need is a cooking method and a good blender. You can start simple and then choose more complex recipes as your comfort level and interest grow along with your baby. And remember, you can always combine single-ingredient purees to make a more elaborate meal.

Most puree recipes follow these three steps:

1. Wash and clean your fruit, vegetable, grain, or meat.

2. Cook foods until soft, using an oven, stovetop steamer or rice cooker, or microwave.

3. Blend to desired texture and use or store for the future.

Choking Hazards

The following foods can present choking hazards and should remain a concern until baby is 4 years old. When you are introducing purees, these are not a problem, as the food will be processed to a smooth texture by your blender or food processor. Nuts and seeds are wonderful additions to pureed foods because they add fat, protein, and fiber, along with many micronutrients. Refer to this list as needed during the food-introduction process.

- Whole nuts and hard seeds
- Hot dogs
- Whole grapes, grape tomatoes, cherry tomatoes
- Hard, gooey, and stick candy, including taffy, gum, and marshmallows
- Certain raw vegetables and fruits, including carrots and apples
- Chunks of nut or seed butter
- Chunks of meat or cheese
- Raisins and dried cranberries
- Fish with bones
- Popcorn

HELPFUL TOOLS AND EQUIPMENT

You do not need complex equipment to make homemade baby food. In fact, you probably have everything required right in your kitchen.

COOKING TOOLS

The recipes in this book are simple and straightforward, and your cooking tools can be, too. If you have a single saucepan and a potato masher, you're all set. Here are some other equipment and appliances that might make this journey a bit easier:

- **MICROWAVE OVEN**

- **SLOTTED SPOON**

- **STEAMER:** Insert for a pan or microwave steamer

- **BASIC POTS AND PANS:** Small (1 quart), medium (3 quart), and large (8 quart)

- **MINI ICE-POP MOLDS:** Teething children love ice pops; so do toddlers, older kids, and adults!

- **MUFFIN TINS:** Whether you choose full-size muffins or miniature, it's good to have these for breakfasts or snacks; most tins are 8- or 12-cup.

- **MEAT THERMOMETER:** This protects flavor and texture, and ensures safety.

- **ELECTRIC PRESSURE COOKER, RICE COOKER, OR SLOW COOKER**

- **A TRADITIONAL OR IMMERSION BLENDER**

STORAGE EQUIPMENT

There are so many options for storing your baby food, but the goal is always convenience and safety. Many people love freezing purees in a silicone ice cube tray. You simply make your puree, freeze it for 6 hours to overnight, then pop out the frozen cubes and store in an airtight container. You then remove and defrost the cubes as needed.

Homemade purees can stay in the refrigerator for 48 to 72 hours and in the freezer for a maximum of 3 months. Be sure to cool any hot purees first by refrigerating for 2 to 3 hours prior to freezing.

For soft items that baby might be trying, such as bananas, avocados, and other soft fruits, consider using a produce-saver storage container. These may seem like an unnecessary expense at first, but they earn their keep when you consider all the berries you may have had to toss out after only one or two days.

FEEDING ESSENTIALS

Parenting isn't easy, so let's keep this simple. Throughout these chapters, I'll be listing stage-specific tools, but there are some tools you will use throughout the food-introduction period and well into toddlerhood.

A SOFT-TIPPED SPOON: This is essential for safely feeding baby a puree. When choosing baby-led feeding, opt for a spoon designed for self-feeding. This type of spoon has a wider grip and often a shorter handle. When spoon-feeding, you will likely need one spoon for yourself and one for baby to hold. My favorite brands include:

- Constructive Eating spoon and fork
- Nuk Gerber Graduates utensils
- The First Years take-and-toss fork
- NumNum GOOtensil; it doubles as a teether
- Pick-Ease, a safe toothpick

WELL-MADE, COLORFUL PLATES AND CUPS: It's best to guide your child away from preferring separated foods, and you can do this by using a non-segmented plate. This may not be possible for a child with a certain level of sensory-processing challenges, and in that case you should follow the direction of your feeding specialist.

THE RIGHT HIGH CHAIR: A good high chair aligns baby to your own seated height. It allows baby to sit up straight, provides foot support, and offers an overall comfortable position. The ideal high chair puts baby's ankles and hips at a 90-degree angle to the legs.

A SIPPY CUP WITH A SOFT SPOUT: This cup will help your baby transition from the breast or bottle to an open cup. Experiment with an open cup, starting as early as 6 months at the table, and even earlier when playing in the bathtub.

SILICONE ICE CUBE FREEZER TRAYS: These trays are convenient for freezing homemade baby food like purees. They release the cubes easily after freezing and are a breeze to clean.

HOW TO USE THIS BOOK

This book will take you through the various stages of food introduction, from 6 to 18 months and beyond. I am your guide from breast or bottle all the way to Baked Salmon Croquettes (page 90) and Mushroom Burgers (page 136). Stick with me, take a deep breath, and get ready to have a lot of fun.

The recipes that follow are indicated as:

30 MINUTES OR LESS
(preparation and cook time, not including ingredient prep)

DAIRY-FREE

GLUTEN-FREE

NUT-FREE

ONE-PAN

VEGAN

VEGETARIAN

You'll also notice some helpful tips:

- **ADDITION TIP:** Suggestions for additions to improve the flavor, texture, or general appeal of a dish.

- **COOKING TIP:** Helps you maximize your time and space while preparing meals.

- **FLAVOR TIP:** Helps you boost your dish by bumping up the flavor.

- **MAKE-AHEAD TIP:** Helps you streamline the cooking process by planning ahead.

- **MEAL TIP:** Suggestions of other recipes and pairings to make a full meal.

- **NUTRITION TIP:** Indicates ways to easily increase the nutrition in a recipe.

- **STORAGE TIP:** Helps you store your food safely for both taste and convenience.

- **SUBSTITUTION TIP:** Guides you toward helpful substitutions in case of allergies, ingredient availability, or flavor preference.

- **TEXTURE TIP:** Presents an opportunity for increased texture exposure.

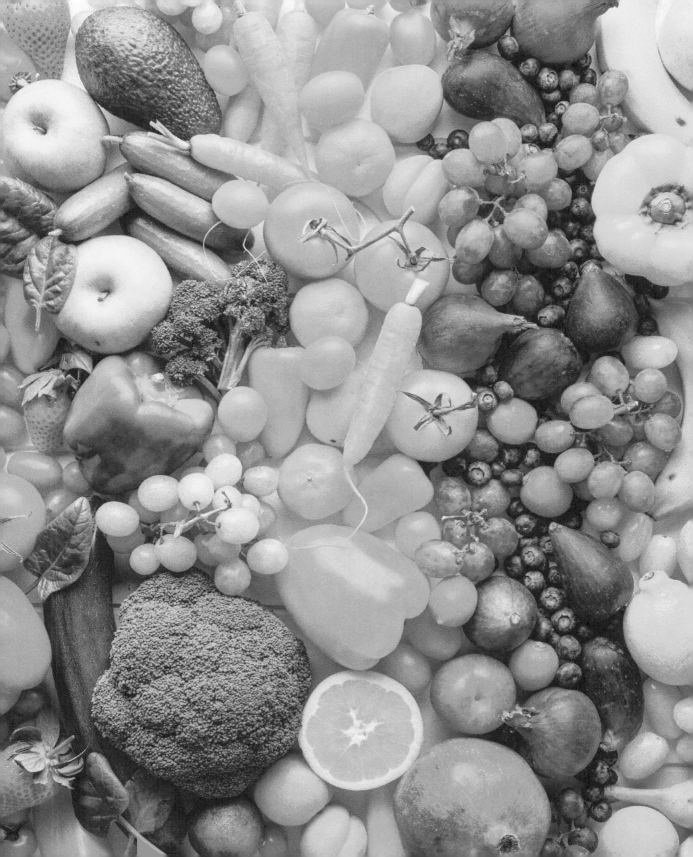

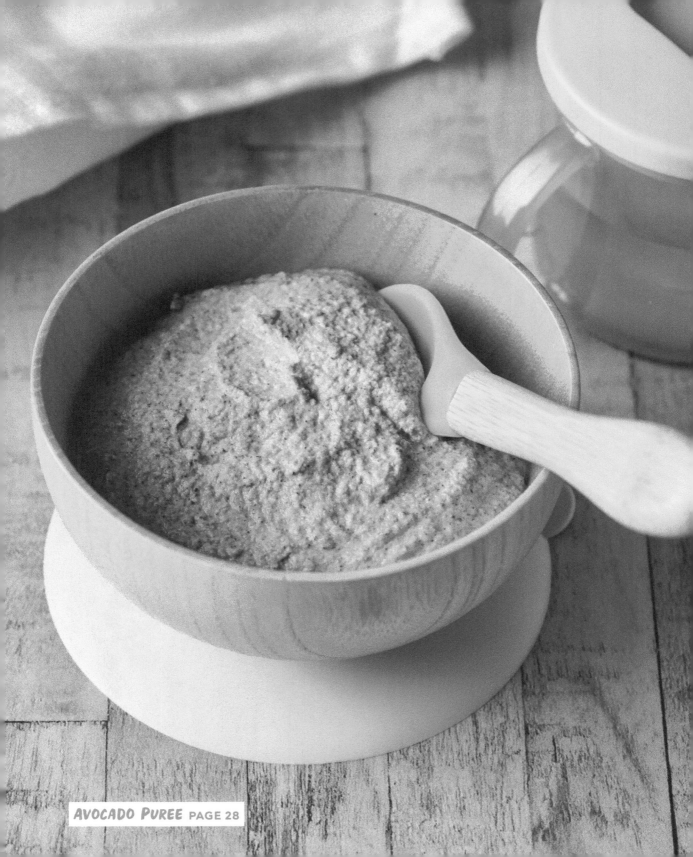

AVOCADO PUREE PAGE 28

2

APPROXIMATELY 6 MONTHS

SINGLE-INGREDIENT PUREES

STARTING STRONG

By 6 months old, your baby has watched you enjoy your meals, hearing the sounds and smelling the smells associated with family dinner—an event they are now, or will soon be, ready to enjoy along with the adults they love. Refer to page 2 for signs that your baby is ready for solids.

This chapter will help you begin your baby's food introduction with confidence. When you can sit with your child and enjoy this moment together, when you can have a moment of peace, a moment when you *know* you are doing the right thing as a parent, that is truly the first step in food introduction.

BABY'S FIRST FOOD

Parents often feel they need to be in control of baby's every moment. That feeling comes with a lot of pressure! Take a deep breath and consider that your child will be the one who truly decides what their first food will be. You can offer, but it's up to baby to indicate whether they are interested. My littlest one didn't want to try anything until the third attempt at food introduction. That's okay! Offering a variety of food, including foods rich in iron and zinc, will help baby meet their needs—even if just a small amount makes it into their belly.

WATCH FOR REACTIONS

This is where responsive feeding comes in. According to the American Academy of Pediatrics (AAP), *responsive feeding* occurs when you pay attention to the signs your baby gives you, allowing their basic biological cues to direct whether they eat and, if so, how much. You may have been advised to feed breast milk or formula on demand. This is a continuation of that theory.

When presented with food, a baby will either lean forward with an open mouth, indicating curiosity, or will turn away. The child who turns away is saying either they are not interested in that food or they are not yet ready for solid food. Any reaction your baby gives is perfectly fine; your role is to listen to what your baby is telling you and respect the cues.

Note: Food reactions that include coughing, wheezing, or swollen lips, tongue, or throat should be addressed immediately. Allergic reactions can become more severe with each new exposure to the allergen, so it's vital that you discuss any reactions with your doctor (see page 6).

Reactions such as constipation or diarrhea are normal and are an expected part of the transition to solid food. These should last only a few days and can be alleviated by blending expressed breast milk into the food, by using a probiotic, or, for alleviating constipation, offering 4 tablespoons (¼ cup) of pure prune or pear juice. Symptoms of food intolerance include gas, constipation, diarrhea, nausea, and headaches. These are often delayed reactions, presenting after a day or even a couple of days. If you suspect your baby is reacting to a particular food, discuss it with your pediatric dietitian.

OPTIMAL NUTRITION

Introduce your baby to different kinds of foods, making them familiar with as many flavors and nutrients as possible and showing your baby that the table is a safe and enjoyable place where you can spend delicious time together.

MAINTAINING BREAST MILK OR FORMULA

Food introduction is important for many reasons, but nutrition still comes from breast milk or formula until the 12-month mark. Breast milk or formula should be served before the meal to ensure that baby isn't overly hungry, a feeling that can derail a well-intended food experience. As your baby grows, you can space the liquid nutrition and solid foods farther apart, making room for appetite to grow while maintaining the nutrition your baby needs. At every stage of this process, I present schedule options to make this as easy as possible for all involved!

All formulas sold in the United States must meet safety and nutrition criteria. If your baby has no gastrointestinal concerns and no painful gas, recurrent diaper or oral rashes, blood in the diaper, congestion, or wheezing, you can feel confident using a standard formula. If your baby is showing signs of an allergy or intolerance, discuss this matter with your pediatric dietitian or pediatrician. You may be directed to a soy formula or another specialty product. When a child reacts to a particular formula, they are usually rejecting the protein in the formula. For babies who appear to react to standard and soy formulas, a doctor may recommend a fully hydrolyzed formula such as Similac Alimentum or Enfamil Nutramigen. Try any new formula for 7 to 10 days before switching to another, so as to give baby time to adjust.

IMPORTANT NUTRIENTS

The only nutrients your baby needs that aren't found in breast milk or formula are zinc and vitamin D. Iron is not found in meaningful quantities in breast milk, but it is added to many formulas. While vitamin D supplementation is strongly recommended by the AAP (see page 101), zinc and iron can be found in many foods.

Good sources of iron include:

- Liver
- Red meat
- Beans, such as red kidney beans, edamame, and chickpeas (garbanzo beans)
- Nuts
- Dried fruits, such as dried apricots
- Fortified breakfast cereals, including baby oatmeal

Good sources of zinc include:

- Shellfish
- Beef
- Pork
- Dairy
- Fortified cereals, including baby oatmeal
- Cashews
- Chickpeas (garbanzo beans)

The best way to ensure adequate nutrition for your baby is to offer a variety of foods. Even the healthiest foods become less than stellar when served on a daily basis. Babies who are just learning how to eat need exposure to different foods for variety in texture and flavor, as well as for nutrition. These different foods provide unique benefits, so it's best to vary the foods offered from day to day or week to week. Switch them up for nutrition, exposure, and overall satisfaction.

FOODS TO EMBRACE

This is a golden moment. Everything you enjoy with your baby is new and exciting to baby. From now until your baby takes that first step is the food-exposure window of opportunity. Think about all the flavors you want your baby to enjoy with you—those Moroccan chickpeas your grandmother made or that spanakopita you savored with your father. Use those connections as goalposts and fill your baby's meals with those delectable memories, using each food experience as a building block toward a lifetime of food enjoyment.

FOODS TO WAIT ON

Not all foods are meant for little ones. Honey carries a risk of botulism that a baby's system may not be able to fight. For that reason, honey, even in cooked products, should be avoided until the 1-year mark.

Also, a baby's kidneys are not mature enough to process the amount of salt that an adult may prefer. Until 1 year, your baby's food should be free of added salt whenever possible. Sodium is a necessary nutrient, but we get enough from whole foods without adding the salt shaker to the table. Instead of salt for flavoring, try salt-free seasonings or herb blends.

TYPICAL TOOLS AND UTENSILS

By choosing high-quality products, you'll be able to use the same utensils as your baby grows. You can also feel confident in keeping preparations simple. You need only the few key essentials listed on page 11. If your child is working with a feeding specialist, check with that person before making your final selections.

When possible, use environmentally friendly products or reuse plastic hand-me-down baby utensils.

TYPICAL MEALS AND SCHEDULE

While it's important to feed your infant on demand, as your baby grows it important to establish a schedule, as babies thrive on predictability. A schedule will help maximize sleep, nutrition—and also your own patience.

At 6 months, your baby is taking three or even four naps per day. Baby is awake for no more than two hours between naps, and sticks to a routine of eat, sleep, and play. Your schedule might look something like the chart on page 20, though it doesn't have to match exactly—check the Resources (page 154) for more information on scheduling.

Sample Meal Schedule

6:00 A.M.	Wake and feed (breast milk or formula)
7:30 A.M.	Solid food breakfast
8:00 A.M.	Morning nap (45 to 60 minutes or more)
9:30 A.M.	Wake and feed (breast milk or formula)
10:00 A.M.	Snack 1
11:00 A.M.	Nap (1½ to 2 hours or more)
1:00 P.M.	Wake and feed (breast milk or formula)
1:30 P.M.	Snack 2
3:00 P.M.	Short nap (20 to 60 minutes)
4:00 P.M.	Wake and feed (breast milk or formula)
4:30 P.M.	Solid food dinner
5:30 P.M.	Begin bedtime routine
6:00 P.M.	Breast milk or formula, then to bed

COMMON CHALLENGES

Here are some common challenges at this stage.

ALLERGIES

As stated earlier, food allergies are much less common than you might believe. If your family does have a history of food allergies, it's best to introduce one food at a time, separating the introductions of new foods by three days. High-allergen foods, like The Big 8 (see page 6), should be introduced even more slowly, with 7 days between new foods. If there is no significant family history of food allergies, though, you can feel confident proceeding at a faster clip, giving your baby new foods as your family enjoys them. Keep in mind that babies generally don't inherit specific food allergies, but they might inherit a propensity to have a *reaction* to a food. For example, if a parent is allergic to shellfish, the child is more likely to be allergic to a food, but not to shellfish specifically.

CONSTIPATION

A healthy baby will have at least one well-formed bowel movement per day, but at the start of solid-food introduction, there is often a short period of adjustment. Monitor baby for straining and crying during bowel movements, lack of appetite, or refusal to eat, a hard belly, hard pellets in the diaper, or streaks of blood in the stool. If constipation lasts longer than a few days, try these gentle methods to help things along:

1. **LOOK FOR PATTERNS:** Constipation may indicate a food sensitivity.

2. **LOWER THE IRON LEVEL:** A high level of iron can cause constipation. Consider switching out iron-fortified foods for non-fortified versions.

3. **PUSH THE P'S:** Pears, plums, peaches, and prunes are known for helping with constipation. Avoid BRAT foods (bananas, rice, applesauce, and toast) during this time.

4. **TUMMY TIME:** Tummy-time activities will help move things along. You can make this more engaging by surrounding your baby with some favorite toys. Tummy time should last three to five minutes, two to three times per day.

5. **TUMMY MASSAGE:** Give your baby an infant massage for constipation. Check out kristyscottage.com/tummy-massage-for-baby for instructions, with helpful pictures.

6. **BABYWEARING:** The combination of your baby's position in the carrier and the skin-to-skin contact puts them in the best position to help mobilize the tummy.

7. **CHIROPRACTIC CARE:** Find a chiropractor who specializes in infant/baby care.

8. **PROBIOTICS:** Look for a refrigerated powder containing at least four species or strains of bacteria, including *Lactobacillus* and *Bifidobacterium*. Following package instructions, mix a small amount into expressed breast milk, prepared formula, or water, and give orally by syringe to the baby. My favorite probiotic for this age is Klaire Labs for Infants.

9. **JUICE:** Try 4 tablespoons (¼ cup) of 100 percent prune or pear juice. While I don't advocate juice as part of a baby's daily diet, these juices have proven to be successful for this medical purpose.

Storage Tips for All Purees

TO REFRIGERATE: Store in a sealed container in the refrigerator for up to 5 days.

TO FREEZE: Portion into ice cube trays or a silicone baby-food freezer tray. Freeze, then release the cubes and store in an airtight container for up to 3 months, removing cubes as needed.

TO THAW: Defrost in one of three ways:

1. Let the puree thaw overnight in the refrigerator.
2. Place sealed bags of frozen puree in a warm-water bath until thawed.
3. Place frozen baby food in a microwave-safe dish and use the defrost function to thaw. Stir frequently and be sure the food is the appropriate temperature prior to serving.

TO SERVE: Serve thawed baby food within 48 hours of defrosting. Discard any food that remains beyond that time.

MIXED BERRY PUREE

30 MINUTES OR LESS | **DAIRY-FREE** | **GLUTEN-FREE** | **NUT-FREE** | **VEGAN**

YIELD: 4 (2-ounce/¼-cup) servings **PREP TIME:** 10 minutes **COOK TIME:** 5 minutes

1 cup mixed fresh
or frozen berries
1 to 4 tablespoons
water
3 tablespoons
water, breast milk,
or formula

Berries are nutritious and flavorful. You can use either fresh or frozen for this puree. Frozen fruit is often more cost-effective and can actually be higher in nutrition, as it's picked at the peak of ripeness and immediately frozen. Fresh fruit is picked before it fully ripens and then travels a long distance to your grocery shelf.

1. In a small saucepan, combine the berries and 1 tablespoon water.

2. Simmer over medium heat for 5 minutes to allow the berries to break down. Watch closely to avoid burning. Add more water, about 1 tablespoon at a time, as needed.

3. Once the berries are broken down, add the 3 tablespoons water, breast milk, or formula, and transfer to a blender or food processor. Blend until smooth.

4. Press the mixture through a fine-mesh sieve by using the back of a spoon, then discard the seeds.

MEAL TIP: Mix the puree with yogurt, oatmeal, or cottage cheese; serve as a dip for toast or banana or pear slices as your baby progresses to finger foods.

MELON PUREE

30 MINUTES OR LESS · DAIRY-FREE · **NUT-FREE** · VEGAN

YIELD: 4 (2-ounce/¼-cup) servings   **PREP TIME:** 5 minutes

1 cup diced fresh melon, any seeds removed

2 tablespoons water, breast milk, or formula, as needed

2 tablespoons oat flour, as needed

I love playing "Melon Roulette" with my kids. We buy an unfamiliar melon and see who can guess what color it is inside. Until your children are old enough to participate in that game, they can enjoy this melon puree. Use any melon you like; just keep in mind that each type of melon will have a different water content.

Blend the melon in a blender or food processor. If it's too thick, add the water, breast milk, or formula; if too thin, add the oat flour 1 teaspoon at a time until you reach the desired consistency.

NUTRITION TIP: Cantaloupe is a surprising source of folate, which is a B vitamin that is essential in brain development and function.

ROASTED BANANA PUREE

30 MINUTES OR LESS | **DAIRY-FREE** | **GLUTEN-FREE** | **NUT-FREE** | **VEGAN**

YIELD: 8 (2-ounce/¼-cup) servings **PREP TIME:** 5 minutes **COOK TIME:** 10 to 12 minutes

Nonstick cooking
  spray (optional)
4 medium bananas,
  peeled and cut
  lengthwise

Bananas are the ultimate classic baby food. Roasting them enhances their flavor and softens them. Combine this puree with oatmeal for a delicious meal or wait until the baby is sleeping and eat it yourself on top of ice cream!

1. Preheat the oven to 350°F. Line a baking sheet with parchment paper or use aluminum foil and coat with cooking spray.

2. Lay the bananas on the baking sheet and roast until golden brown, 10 to 12 minutes.

3. Place the bananas in a blender or food processor and blend for 1 to 2 minutes, to the desired consistency.

4. Cool and serve, or store in the freezer for later use.

FLAVOR TIP: Add seasonings to boost flavor exposure, such as ⅛ teaspoon chopped fresh rosemary, ½ teaspoon ground cinnamon, ¼ teaspoon ground cloves, ¼ teaspoon ground nutmeg, or ¼ teaspoon grated fresh ginger!

PEACH PUREE

DAIRY-FREE GLUTEN-FREE NUT-FREE VEGAN

YIELD: 8 (2-ounce/¼-cup) servings **PREP TIME:** 5 to 10 minutes, plus 10 minutes to cool
COOK TIME: 20 to 25 minutes

Nonstick cooking
  spray (optional)
2 pounds (about
  6 medium) fresh
  peaches, peeled,
  pitted, and sliced,
  or 1 pound frozen
  peach slices

Peaches have a vibrant flavor and creamy texture that your baby is sure to love. Peaches, along with pears and plums, are known for their ability to help with constipation.

1. Preheat the oven to 425°F. Line a baking sheet with parchment paper or use aluminum foil and coat with cooking spray.

2. Place the peach slices in one layer on the baking sheet. Roast for 20 to 25 minutes, until the edges begin to caramelize.

3. Remove from the oven and let cool for 10 minutes.

4. Place the peaches in a blender or food processor and blend for 1 to 2 minutes, to desired consistency.

5. Cool and serve, or store in the freezer for up to 3 months.

FLAVOR TIP: Add a pinch of ground cinnamon prior to roasting!

NUTRITION TIP: Pair the peach puree with applesauce, oatmeal, or sweet potato puree to enhance the nutritional profile.

DRIED APRICOT PUREE

DAIRY-FREE GLUTEN-FREE NUT-FREE VEGAN

YIELD: 10 (2-ounce/¼-cup) servings **PREP TIME:** 2 minutes, plus 2 to 3 hours to soak
COOK TIME: 2 minutes

2 cups water
½ cup unsulphured
   dried apricots
1 to 2 tablespoons
   water, breast milk,
   or formula

Dried fruit can be a good source of iron—one of the few nutrients that are meaningful in baby's food at this time. This puree can also be made with prunes! Both prunes and apricots are beneficial if your baby is constipated (see page 21).

1. In a small pot or bowl, bring the water to a boil, then turn off the heat. Add the apricots, cover, and let sit for 2 to 3 hours, or until soft.

2. Place the apricots and water in a blender or food processor and blend until smooth. Add 1 to 2 tablespoons water, breast milk, or formula as needed for the desired texture.

FLAVOR TIP: Some dried apricots can be a bit bitter, so this puree should be paired with another sweet puree, such as banana, or mixed with yogurt or oatmeal.

AVOCADO PUREE

30 MINUTES OR LESS | **DAIRY-FREE** | **GLUTEN-FREE** | **NUT-FREE** | **VEGAN**

YIELD: 2 or 3 (2-ounce/¼-cup) servings **PREP TIME:** 5 minutes

1 Hass avocado
2 tablespoons
   water, breast milk,
   or formula

Avocados are an amazing fat source, and fat is essential for brain development during these tender years. Avocados are versatile and provide such a great opportunity for color exposure!

1. Scoop out and cut the avocado into rough chunks.

2. Place the chunks in a blender or food processor and blend along with the water, breast milk, or formula to the desired consistency.

STORAGE TIP: Refrigerate this puree in a container with the avocado pit to keep the color bright and taste fresh.
   If freezing, be sure to store in an airtight container. You can actually freeze whole avocados! If you're not quite ready to use an avocado you just purchased, wrap it tightly in foil and store in the freezer until the mood strikes, up to 3 months.

ROASTED BUTTERNUT SQUASH PUREE

DAIRY-FREE GLUTEN-FREE NUT-FREE VEGAN

YIELD: 16 (2-ounce/¼-cup) servings **PREP TIME:** 10 minutes, plus 30 minutes to cool
COOK TIME: 60 to 80 minutes

Nonstick cooking
  spray (optional)
1 medium
  butternut squash
  (2 to 3 pounds),
  washed, or
  4½ cups cubed
  fresh squash,
  or 1 (14-ounce)
  bag frozen
  squash cubes
2 tablespoons
  water, breast milk,
  or formula

The most challenging part of cooking with a butternut squash is cutting into it. So, let's just skip that step by roasting it whole! Alternatively, use pre-cut squash or bags of frozen squash cubes.

1. Preheat the oven to 425°F. Line a half-sheet pan with parchment paper or use aluminum foil and lightly coat with cooking spray.

2. Pierce the squash in 5 or 6 places with a sharp knife.

3. Place the squash on the sheet pan. Roast for 60 to 80 minutes, until a knife goes in easily. Note: It will be brown and a bit shriveled.

4. Let the squash cool completely, about 30 minutes.

5. Slice the squash in half lengthwise, scoop out the seeds, and peel off the brown skin.

6. Place the flesh in a blender or food processor. Blend to desired consistency, adding the water, breast milk, or formula as needed.

FLAVOR TIP: Kick up the flavor by adding 1 teaspoon chopped fresh thyme to the blender or food processor.

NUTRITION TIP: One cup of butternut squash provides a powerful punch of nutrition:100 percent of vitamin A, 40 percent of vitamin C, and 18 percent of your daily potassium!

SPRING PEA PUREE

30 MINUTES OR LESS **DAIRY-FREE** **GLUTEN-FREE** **NUT-FREE** **VEGAN**

YIELD: 8 (2-ounce/¼-cup) servings **PREP TIME:** 5 minutes **COOKING TIME:** 2 to 4 minutes

2 cups frozen peas
3 tablespoons
water, breast milk,
or formula

Did you know that the Romans grew over 37 varieties of peas? And Queen Elizabeth I had peas shipped to England to be sure she could enjoy them? Also, the first television commercial aired in color was an advertisement for frozen peas! Enjoy this bright green puree, which is vibrant in both color and nutrition.

1. Thaw the peas by steaming them for 3 minutes in the microwave or 2 to 4 minutes in a saucepan on the stovetop.

2. Place the peas in a blender or food processor along with the water, breast milk, or formula and blend to the desired consistency.

NUTRITION TIP: Just under 1 cup of peas provides more protein than a whole egg!

CARROT PUREE

DAIRY-FREE **GLUTEN-FREE** **NUT-FREE** **ONE PAN** **VEGAN**

YIELD: 5 (2-ounce/¼-cup) servings **PREP TIME:** 5 minutes, plus 20 minutes to cool
COOK TIME: 20 minutes

1 pound carrots
   (about 5 medium),
   trimmed
2 tablespoons
   breast milk or
   formula (optional)

Carrots come in a wide array of colors! To make a beautiful puree, stick with one color family, but as soon as you are ready to move beyond purees, introduce your baby—and the rest of the family as well—to the vibrant yellow carrot or the majestic purple carrot, which has a fun surprise in the middle! Mix up your colors and nutrition by adding other root vegetables, such as beets, parsnips, or even daikon.

1. Clean the carrots by peeling the rough outer skin, then chop into ½-inch pieces.

2. Bring a medium saucepan of water to a boil over high heat. Add the carrots and boil for 20 minutes, or until tender enough to pierce with a knife.

3. Remove the carrots from water, reserving at least 2 tablespoons of the cooking liquid, and allow to cool for 20 minutes.

4. Put the carrots in a blender or food processor, adding either the reserved cooking liquid or the breast milk or formula, and blend to desired consistency, adding more liquid as needed.

NUTRITION TIP: Carrots are high in antioxidants, which help support immune health.

SWEET POTATO PUREE

DAIRY-FREE GLUTEN-FREE NUT-FREE VEGAN

YIELD: 8 (2-ounce/¼-cup) servings **PREP TIME:** 5 minutes, plus 30 minutes to cool
COOK TIME: 45 to 50 minutes

Nonstick cooking
  spray (optional)
4 medium sweet
  potatoes,
  scrubbed well
2 tablespoons
  water, breast milk,
  or formula, plus
  more as needed

True yams are a different root vegetable from sweet potatoes, though the names are often used interchangeably. A true yam is very large, fibrous, and brown-skinned; it is less common because it comes from Africa and Latin America, whereas sweet potatoes are grown in the southern United States. The sweet potato is long and tapered, and is soft and sweet when cooked. There are many different types of sweet potatoes, including white, purple, and—the most common—orange. Try using different varieties of sweet potato for increased exposure for both your baby and the rest of your family!

1. Preheat the oven to 425°F. Line a baking sheet with parchment paper or use aluminum foil and coat with cooking spray.

2. Poke 4 or 5 holes in each sweet potato and place on the baking sheet. Bake for 45 to 50 minutes, or until tender.

3. Let cool for 30 minutes.

4. Scrape out the flesh of the sweet potatoes, place in a blender or food processor along with the water, breast milk, or formula, and blend to desired consistency, adding a tablespoon or more liquid as needed for texture.

MEAL TIP: Sweet potato puree, much like traditional mashed potatoes, can be a delicious side dish long after initial food introduction. Enjoy it alongside your favorite meals as your baby grows!

TRADITIONAL APPLESAUCE

DAIRY-FREE **GLUTEN-FREE** **NUT-FREE** **VEGAN**

YIELD: 8 (2-ounce/¼-cup) servings **PREP TIME:** 5 minutes, plus 15 minutes to cool
COOK TIME: 15 to 20 minutes

2 medium apples,
  peeled if desired,
  seeded, and cored
1 teaspoon lemon
  juice

To peel or not to peel—you can go either way with this simple applesauce. Keeping the peel on the apple can increase fiber, vitamin K, vitamin C, calcium, and potassium. The flesh of an apple has soluble fiber and plenty of phytonutrients. Different varieties of apples will provide a different flavor experience. Try Granny Smith for a tart flavor, Honeycrisp for a traditional sweet sensation, or a mix—any variety of ripe apple will work in this recipe. (Note: This recipe combines nicely with the Sweet Potato Puree on page 32).

1. Roughly chop the apples and add to a small saucepan.

2. Cook over medium heat, stirring regularly to avoid burning, for 15 to 20 minutes, or until tender. The apples will release their natural liquid as they cook down.

3. Add the lemon juice and stir, then turn off the heat. Cool for about 15 minutes.

4. Add the apples to a blender or food processor and blend to the desired consistency.

TEXTURE TIP: As your baby grows and you become more comfortable presenting more textured foods, you can use a potato masher instead of a blender for a thicker and chunkier applesauce.

FLAVOR TIP: Add ¼ teaspoon ground cinnamon to the cooking apples to increase exposure to flavor and smell.

ROASTED BROCCOLI AND OLIVE OIL PUREE

DAIRY-FREE **GLUTEN-FREE** **NUT-FREE** **VEGAN**

YIELD: 6 (2-ounce/¼-cup) servings **PREP TIME:** 10 minutes, plus 15 minutes to cool
COOK TIME: 10 to 12 minutes

Olive oil cooking
  spray
1 pound broccoli
  crowns, cut
  into florets
  and washed
1 tablespoon
  olive oil
2 tablespoons
  water, breast milk,
  formula, tahini,
  or Sweet Potato
  Puree (page 32)

This versatile puree has a wonderful, vibrant color, representing the amazing phytonutrients found in broccoli. Consider allowing your baby to play with a big head of broccoli as you prepare this dish. The many sensory experiences that broccoli can provide are wonderful for food and color exposure, as well as for the development of fine and gross motor skills.

1. Preheat the oven to 425°F. Line a baking sheet with aluminum foil and coat liberally with olive oil spray.

2. Place the florets in a medium bowl, drizzle on the olive oil, and toss to coat each piece.

3. Spread the broccoli on the baking sheet in a single layer. Roast for 10 to 12 minutes, or until completely tender.

4. Remove from the oven and let cool for about 15 minutes.

5. Add the broccoli to a blender or food processor and blend to the desired consistency, adding the water, breast milk, or formula, or even tahini or the sweet potato puree, 1 tablespoon at a time.

NUTRITION TIP: While some babies may have increased gas from eating cruciferous veggies, most will not have a problem. And remember—better out than in! If your baby is expelling that gas effectively, keep going! If you do believe that your little one is struggling to expel gas, you can always return to cruciferous vegetables in another month, when your baby's digestive tract is more developed.

STEAMED GREEN BEAN PUREE

30 MINUTES OR LESS | DAIRY-FREE | GLUTEN-FREE | NUT-FREE | VEGAN

YIELD: 6 (2-ounce/¼-cup) servings **PREP TIME:** 5 to 10 minutes **COOK TIME:** 2 to 5 minutes

1 pound fresh green beans, trimmed and sliced, or 1 (12-ounce) bag frozen green beans

2 tablespoons breast milk or formula (optional)

Every year when I was growing up, on Thanksgiving I would watch the Macy's Thanksgiving Day Parade with my mom. Now, I get to watch with my kids. The Jolly Green Giant balloon never ceases to amaze me. It can be so much fun to relate our favorite foods to fun characters and enjoyable family time.

1. Using a stovetop or microwave steamer, steam the fresh beans for 3 to 5 minutes or the frozen for 2 to 3 minutes.

2. Remove the beans from the steamer and rinse with cold water to cool. Reserve 2 tablespoons of the cooking water.

3. Place the beans in a blender or food processor and blend to desired consistency, adding either the reserved cooking water or the breast milk or formula, as needed, 1 tablespoon at a time.

NUTRITION TIP: To increase flavor and nutrition, consider adding 1 tablespoon chopped fresh basil to the blender or food processor in step 3. Basil contains vitamin K, which is great for bone health, and manganese, essential for proper utilization of many other nutrients!

SPINACH PUREE

30 MINUTES OR LESS DAIRY-FREE GLUTEN-FREE NUT-FREE VEGAN

YIELD: 4 (2-ounce/¼-cup) servings **PREP TIME:** 10 minutes **COOK TIME:** 2 to 5 minutes

6 cups (packed) trimmed fresh spinach, or 2 cups frozen chopped spinach
2 tablespoons breast milk or formula (optional)

Spinach can have a bitter flavor undertone that makes it unappealing to some toddlers. Babies, on the other hand, have super-sensitive taste buds and can appreciate the depth of flavor spinach provides. By exposing your child to this flavor profile early on, they are more likely to continue to enjoy it and avoid that food neophobia phase.

1. Wash the fresh spinach well, then dry by patting it with a dish towel or spinning it in a salad spinner.

2. Using a stovetop or microwave steamer, steam the fresh spinach for 3 to 5 minutes or until wilted; if using frozen spinach, steam for 2 to 3 minutes.

3. Remove spinach from the steamer and immediately run under cold water to stop the cooking, then drain. Reserve 2 tablespoons of the cooking liquid.

4. Place the spinach in a blender or food processor and blend to desired consistency, adding either the reserved cooking liquid or the breast milk or formula, 1 tablespoon at a time.

MEAL TIP: If this puree isn't accepted by your baby as it is, consider pairing it with Traditional Applesauce (page 33), Sweet Potato Puree (page 32), or Bean Puree (page 40). You can also add the spinach puree to muffin batter, include it in soups, or use it as a base to create a savory sauce!

SLOW COOKER CHICKEN PUREE

DAIRY-FREE GLUTEN-FREE NUT-FREE

YIELD: 4 (2-ounce/¼-cup) servings **PREP TIME:** 5 minutes, plus 10 to 15 minutes to cool
COOK TIME: 4 to 6 hours, unattended

2 cups low- or
  no-sodium
  chicken or
  vegetable broth
2½ pounds
  assorted skinless
  chicken pieces
  with bone
Seasonings of
  choice (see
  Nutrition Tip)

The simplest way to make baby food is to blend what the rest of the family is eating as solid food! This easy slow cooker chicken recipe is sure to please your little one, while also providing dinner for the rest of the family. Add any seasonings your family enjoys, but add just minimal salt, as your baby's kidneys are not yet developed enough to handle an adult serving of sodium.

1. Pour the broth into the slow cooker.

2. Layer the chicken pieces on top. Add seasonings as desired, cover, and slow-cook for 4 hours on high or for 6 hours on low.

3. If necessary, switch the setting to keep the rest of the chicken warm, then remove the chicken piece intended for baby. Let it cool for 10 to 15 minutes.

4. Separate the meat from the bone. Place the meat in a food processor or blender and blend to desired consistency, adding some of the cooking liquid, 1 tablespoon at a time, as needed.

NUTRITION TIP: Boost the nutrition and flavor by adding ½ large onion, chopped, to the cooking broth; sprinkle on the chicken 1 tablespoon diced garlic, 3 fresh basil leaves or 1 teaspoon dried basil, 1 teaspoon dried oregano, 1 teaspoon ground cumin, and/or 1 teaspoon sweet or smoked paprika.

BEEF PUREE

`DAIRY-FREE` `GLUTEN-FREE` `NUT-FREE`

YIELD: 6 (2-ounce/¼-cup) servings **PREP TIME:** 10 minutes, plus 10 minutes to cool
COOK TIME: 25 minutes

8 ounces boneless sirloin beef (or top round, chuck, or flank steak)

2 cups low- or no-sodium beef or vegetable broth

Meat is often overlooked as a first-food option. If your family enjoys eating meat, your baby can, too. Timing is essential on this, however, because waiting too long after cooking to puree will yield tough meat that won't blend well. Note: This recipe is the simplest method for making a beef puree.

1. Cut the meat into cubes, discarding any gristle or unwanted fat. (Fat is important for your baby's brain development, so don't toss it all!)

2. Pour the broth into a medium saucepan and bring to a boil over high heat. Add the meat, then reduce the heat to a low simmer. Simmer for 20 minutes, until the meat is tender and reaches an internal temperature of 145°F.

3. Allow the meat and broth to cool together for about 10 minutes.

4. Using a slotted spoon, transfer the meat to a blender or food processor. Reserve 2 tablespoons of the cooking liquid.

5. Blend to desired consistency, slowly adding the reserved cooking liquid as needed.

NUTRITION TIP: Meat provides protein, iron, and B vitamins, which are important for growth and development.

PAPAYA PUREE

30 MINUTES OR LESS | DAIRY-FREE | GLUTEN-FREE | NUT-FREE | VEGAN

YIELD: 6 (2-ounce/¼-cup) servings **PREP TIME:** 10 minutes

1 ripe medium
   papaya, or
   12 ounces frozen
   papaya, partially
   thawed
2 tablespoons
   water, breast milk,
   or formula

Need to get away to someplace warm? A tropical puree can take you there! This delicious recipe can be expanded to be a meal when served with oatmeal, yogurt, or cottage cheese. The puree can also be frozen into mini ice pops for a great teething option.

1. Wash the papaya, then slice it lengthwise.

2. Remove the seeds and scoop out the papaya flesh.

3. Place the flesh in a blender or food processor and blend to desired consistency, adding the water, breast milk, or formula as needed, 1 tablespoon at a time.

MEAL TIP: Pair the papaya puree with Roasted Banana Puree (page 25) for a creamy and tropical experience.

BEAN PUREE

30 MINUTES OR LESS | **DAIRY-FREE** | **GLUTEN-FREE** | **NUT-FREE** | **VEGAN**

YIELD: 4 (2-ounce/¼-cup) servings **PREP TIME:** 10 minutes

1 (15-ounce) can
low-sodium black
beans, chickpeas,
white beans,
or any other
desired variety

2 tablespoons
water, breast milk,
or formula

Not only do beans blend to a smooth and creamy consistency, but they are also a natural source of protein, fiber, iron, folate, zinc, calcium, phosphorus, and many B vitamins. And beans pair well with many other purees to create satisfying and well-rounded meals. You can use canned beans or reconstituted dried beans. If using canned, look for "BPA-free lining" on the label and choose no-salt-added brands. If you are reconstituting dried beans, put them in the slow cooker, cover with water (using twice as much water as beans), and cook on high for 3 hours. Drain, rinse, and cool and you're ready to go!

1. Drain the beans and rinse well.

2. Place in a blender or food processor and blend to desired consistency, adding the water, breast milk, or formula as needed, 1 tablespoon at a time.

MEAL TIP: Consider pairing a puree of black beans with blueberry puree (see page 23) or Roasted Banana Puree (page 25). Add white bean puree to Roasted Butternut Squash Puree (page 29). Add a chickpea puree to the Slow Cooker Chicken Puree (page 37).

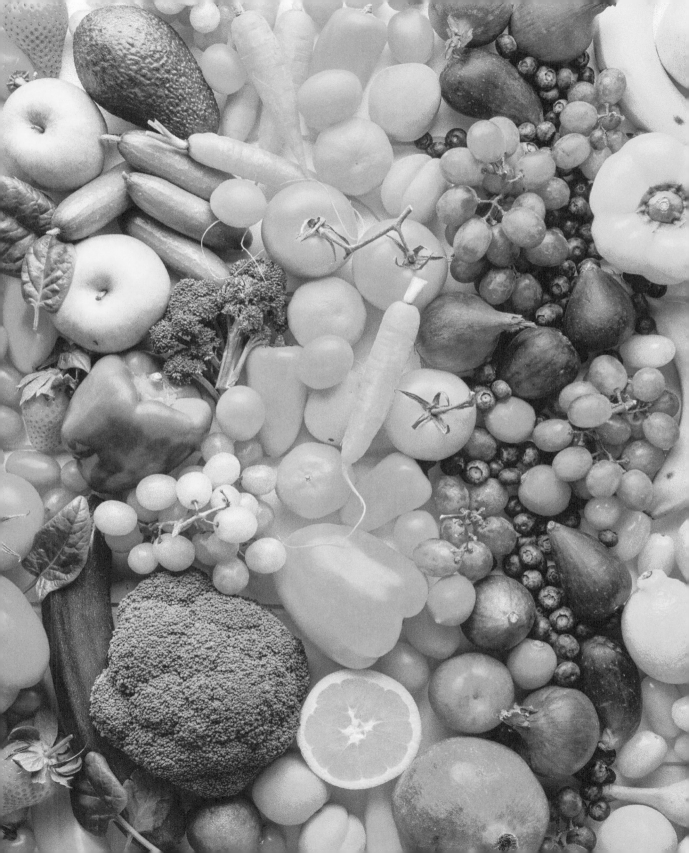

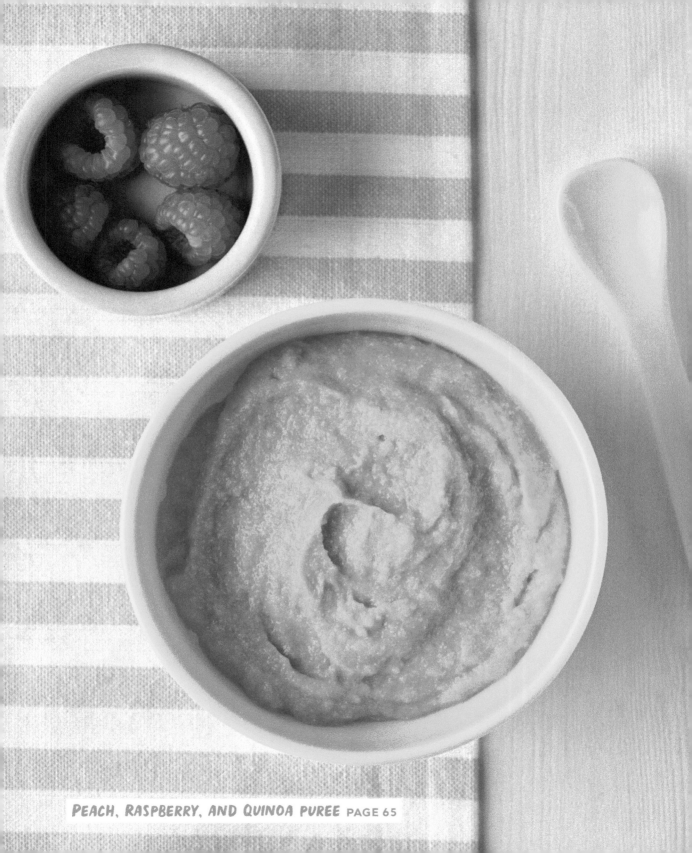

PEACH, RASPBERRY, AND QUINOA PUREE PAGE 65

3

6 TO 8 MONTHS

COMBINATION PUREES

OPTIMAL NUTRITION

Ready to get spicy? Okay, maybe it's not time to introduce your baby to habaneros, but if you haven't been using seasoning or haven't yet been combining flavors in your baby's food, now is the time to start! The foods that become familiar now will be your baby's comfort food in years to come. Take advantage of this opportunity to share your favorite flavors with your little one.

If you were to walk down the baby-food aisle of your local grocery store, you would notice a huge variety of flavors and colors. There is a rhyme to this reason: introducing your baby to many different flavors will set them up for a lifetime of food enjoyment. The sheer amount of choice can be overwhelming, though, so here are some guidelines.

MAINTAINING BREAST MILK OR FORMULA

Until 12 months, breast milk or formula provides ideal nutrition and should continue to be served before any solid meal. As nutritious as spinach, squash, and bananas are, their overall nutrient profile can't compete with breast milk or formula. By serving liquid nutrition before sitting your baby down for a meal, you make sure that their nutrition needs are met while also setting the scene for a happy session of food exploration.

IMPORTANT NUTRIENTS

Just as discussed in chapter 2, the important nutrients coming from your baby's solid-food experience are limited to iron and zinc (see page 18). The rest of their necessary nutritional needs right now are still met with breast milk or formula. Nevertheless, the many sensory experiences provided by the colorful and tasty meals you're preparing for your baby are essential for oral muscle development, as well as familiarization with different flavors, smells, and even sounds. The more food experiences your baby enjoys now, the more they will continue to enjoy as they grow and truly begin to rely on those nutrients.

FOODS TO EMBRACE

Think back to your own favorite food experiences. Is there something from your childhood that you would like to share? A favorite dish from your culture? A fond memory you would like to relive through your baby's wondrous eyes?

Keep these dishes in mind as you progress, working toward presenting them to your baby. Baby food doesn't have to be confined to bland flavors. The food you give your baby should reflect the joyful moments of your own experiences.

FOODS TO WAIT ON

Honey and salt remain foods to avoid until 12 months (see page 19). Your baby can have a small amount of salt, but it's best to avoid adding salt to dishes. Consider using other seasonings to flavor food or relying on your baby's uniquely sensitive taste buds to savor the subtle flavors that adults cannot detect. Honey should be avoided in all forms, even when cooked, until 12 months owing to the risk of infant botulism. At the 12-month mark, your baby's kidneys are stronger and more developed, as is their immune system. They will then be able to process more salt and to fight off infant botulism, should they be exposed to it.

TEETHING CONSIDERATIONS

If your usually happy baby is suddenly inconsolable, it might be due to teething. If your baby is suddenly up at night, they might be teething. If your baby is having trouble nursing or eating, they might be teething. If your baby is suddenly running a fever and has diaper rash, it may be related to teething. All babies react to teething in their own way—some are happy teethers, and others are miserable. Here are some practical tips for coping with this situation:

1. Dip a washcloth in breast milk or formula, freeze it, and give it to your baby for sucking.

2. Make mini ice pops out of breast milk, formula, or a simple recipe like Papaya Puree (page 39).

3. Put small chunks of frozen fruits or vegetables into a mesh teether for your baby.

4. If you're comfortable with baby-led weaning (see page 48), give your baby a frozen waffle or pancake.

If your child isn't into cold foods:

1. Give your baby a big head of raw broccoli to play with. Any amount they are able to bite off will be safe. They will not be able to bite off large chunks.

2. Get some teething oil, like Punkin Butt, for quick, if temporary, relief.

3. Buy a finger toothbrush for massaging your baby's tender gums.

4. Consider a teething toy, such as the Banana Baby Toothbrush, which your baby can manage on their own.

TYPICAL MEALS AND SCHEDULE

On the facing page is a sample schedule for a baby who is 6 to 8 months old. While each baby, and each family, has a different dynamic, finding the schedule that works best for you will make life simpler.

Your baby will continue the established eat, sleep, and play pattern, being awake for no more than two to two and a half hours between naps. You'll know if your schedule isn't working for you if you feel overly anxious about the exact minute your baby falls asleep, if your baby's naps are very short, or if your baby seems out of sorts and not up to playing or exploring. For additional scheduling options, see the Resources (page 154).

Sample Meal Schedule

6:00 A.M.	Wake and feed (breast milk or formula)
7:45 A.M.	Solid food breakfast
8:00 A.M.	Morning nap (45 to 60 minutes or more)
9:30 A.M.	Wake and feed (breast milk or formula)
10:00 A.M.	Snack 1
11:30 A.M.	Nap (1½ to 2 hours or more)
2:00 P.M.	Wake and feed (breast milk or formula)
2:30 P.M.	Snack 2
3:30 P.M.	Short nap (20 to 60 minutes)
5:00 P.M.	Solid food dinner
5:30 P.M.	Begin bedtime routine
6:00 P.M.	Breast milk or formula, then to bed

COMMON CHALLENGES

Here are some common challenges at this age.

BABY DOESN'T SEEM INTERESTED IN FOOD.

There are some reasons this might be happening:

1. **YOUR BABY MIGHT BE TOO YOUNG OR NOT READY FOR SOLIDS.** Check the readiness signs (see page 2) to help determine whether your baby is truly ready for solid food or if you should pull back and wait a little while longer.

2. **YOUR SCHEDULE MIGHT NEED TWEAKING.** Remember, your baby should not have an appetite when they sit down for a meal. At this point, breast milk or formula provides most of the nutrition your little one needs. This is the time to develop feeding skills, which happens through food play and experimentation. Food isn't meant to make their belly full until a bit later on. Be sure to give your baby a bottle or the breast, then explore solid foods with a full belly.

3. **YOU COULD NEED TO MODEL FOOD MORE CLEARLY.** A client came to me with a video of her daughter smearing yogurt all over her body. She didn't seem interested in eating it at all. I asked the mother, "Are you eating it with her?" She answered no. "When was the last time she watched you apply lotion to your body?" Bingo. Modeling is a very important part of learning how to eat. Be sure to enjoy food alongside your child.

4. **MAKE SURE THEIR SEAT IS COMFORTABLE.** Check that their high chair provides 90-degree support at the heels and hips.

5. **GIVE YOUR BABY TIME AND SPACE TO EXPLORE FOOD.** Make time for a slow-paced and fun food experience. Avoid feeding in a rush. At this point, if there isn't time for a slow, enjoyable meal, skip it. Food is for exploration more than nutrition until that 12-month mark.

BABY KEEPS TRYING TO GRAB THE SPOON.

If your baby keeps trying to grab the spoon from you, seems unwilling to accept the spoon from you, or is otherwise being very independent at the table, it might be time to consider a baby-led weaning (BLW) approach. If the thought of putting your baby in charge makes you nervous, consider this: baby-led weaning doesn't necessarily mean giving your baby finger foods. If you're not comfortable with that, you can give purees in a BLW-style, putting your child in the driver's seat while maintaining a feeding dynamic that honors your own concerns. Try these tactics:

1. **GIVE YOUR BABY A SPOON TO HOLD DURING FEEDING.** If your baby is holding a spoon of their own, they may be more willing to accept the food from your spoon.

2. **TRY BLW.** Load up a spoon and simply place it in front of your baby. If your little one is showing all the readiness signs and is interested in food, there is a better than average chance they will pick up the spoon and self-feed.

Storage Tips for All Purees

TO REFRIGERATE: Store in a sealed container in the refrigerator for up to five days.

TO FREEZE: Portion into ice cube trays or a silicone baby-food freezer tray. Freeze, then pop out the cubes and store them in an airtight container for up to 3 months, removing each portion as needed.

TO DEFROST: Defrost in one of three different ways:

1. Let the puree thaw overnight in the refrigerator.
2. Place sealed frozen bags of purees in a warm-water bath until thawed.
3. Place frozen baby food in a microwave-safe dish and use the defrost function on your microwave to thaw. Stir frequently and be sure that the food is the appropriate temperature prior to serving.

TO SERVE: Serve thawed baby food within 48 hours of defrosting. Discard any food that remains beyond that time.

STONE FRUIT SLOW COOKER PUREE

`DAIRY-FREE` `GLUTEN-FREE` `NUT-FREE` `VEGAN`

YIELD: 10 (2-ounce/¼-cup) servings **PREP TIME:** 5 to 10 minutes **COOK TIME:** 5 hours, unattended

5 cups pitted and peeled fresh stone fruit

½ cup water

1 vanilla bean, split in half lengthwise (optional)

This delicious puree can be prepared with any stone fruit—either fresh or frozen—such as plums, peaches, nectarines, and apricots. If your baby is experiencing constipation, which often accompanies food introduction, this recipe is the way to go. Pair the puree with yogurt or oatmeal for added probiotics or fiber.

1. Place the fruit in the slow cooker. Add the water and the vanilla bean (if using).

2. Slow-cook on high for 5 hours, until the fruit is fully softened.

3. Remove the vanilla bean and discard or save for another use.

4. Using either an immersion blender in the cooker pot or transferring to a blender or food processor, puree the fruit to the desired consistency, adding a small amount of the cooking liquid, if necessary, for a smooth mixture.

ADDITION TIP: You can put more zing in this recipe by adding pitted sweet cherries. No need to peel!

COOKING TIP: The exact amount of water needed to puree the fruit depends on which fruit you use. If blending in the cooker itself, pour off any excess water. Alternatively, cook the fruit another hour, uncovered, so some of the liquid can boil off.

CAULIFLOWER AND SPINACH PUREE

30 MINUTES OR LESS | DAIRY-FREE | GLUTEN-FREE | NUT-FREE | VEGAN

YIELD: 10 (2-ounce/¼-cup) servings **PREP TIME:** 5 minutes, plus 5 to 10 minutes to cool
COOK TIME: 4 to 15 minutes

1 head of
cauliflower,
trimmed and cut
into florets
1 garlic clove
2 cups (packed)
fresh baby spinach
About 2 tablespoons
olive oil

You can find cauliflower rice, cauliflower pizza crust, and even cauliflower as a meat replacement! With this recipe, let's enjoy this beautiful vegetable for what it is—delicious, nutritious, creamy, and great for flavor exposure and food enjoyment.

1. Using a stovetop steamer insert or a microwave, steam the cauliflower and garlic until tender, about 15 minutes in a stovetop steamer or 4 to 5 minutes in a microwave.

2. Let cool for 5 to 10 minutes, then place the cauliflower in a blender or food processor. Add handfuls of the spinach and drizzles of oil while blending, until smooth.

MEAL TIP: Serve with Bean Puree (page 40) or Slow Cooker Chicken Puree (page 37) for a well-rounded meal. If the taste is a bit bitter, you can mix in some Traditional Applesauce (page 33).

STRAWBERRY-BANANA PUREE

30 MINUTES OR LESS | **DAIRY-FREE** | **GLUTEN-FREE** | **NUT-FREE** | **VEGAN**

YIELD: 4 (2-ounce/¼-cup) servings **PREP TIME:** 5 minutes

1 medium
  banana, sliced
½ cup hulled
  fresh or frozen
  strawberries
1 tablespoon
  gluten-free oat
  flour (optional)

What is a more classic combination than strawberry and banana? It's the taste of sunshine, of carefree childhood moments. This creamy puree is delicious on its own but can also be served with yogurt or oatmeal.

1. Place the banana and strawberries in a blender or food processor, and blend until smooth.

2. If a thicker texture is desired, blend in the oat flour, 1 teaspoon at a time, until desired consistency is reached.

MEAL TIP: This puree can be a dip for other fruits, or a pancake or waffle topping; alternatively, you can freeze it into ice pops, which are wonderful for teething babies.

MANGO, BANANA, AND SWEET POTATO PUREE

30 MINUTES OR LESS | **DAIRY-FREE** | **GLUTEN-FREE** | **NUT-FREE** | **VEGAN**

YIELD: 12 (2-ounce/¼-cup) servings **PREP TIME:** 5 minutes, plus 10 minutes to cool
COOK TIME: 5 to 15 minutes

1 medium sweet
  potato, peeled
  and chopped
1½ cups chopped
  fresh or frozen
  mango
1 medium banana,
  peeled

Mangos are a creamy and vibrant fruit, high in flavor and vitamin C. They pair nicely with both sweet and savory flavors. If fresh mangos are not available or out of season, you can use frozen mango for this convenient and nutritious meal.

1. Using a stovetop steamer insert or a microwave, steam the sweet potato for 12 to 15 minutes until soft, or microwave on high for 5 to 7 minutes.

2. Allow the sweet potato to cool, about 10 minutes.

3. Place the mango, banana, and sweet potato in a blender or food processor and blend to the desired consistency.

NUTRITION TIP: Bananas can be a binding food, so if your baby has slowed down on the dirty diapers, producing fewer than one bowel movement per day, it's best to avoid bananas, rice, applesauce, and toast (BRAT) until your baby is pooping at least once per day.

BUCKWHEAT AND YOGURT

30 MINUTES OR LESS | GLUTEN-FREE | NUT-FREE | VEGETARIAN

YIELD: 12 (2-ounce/¼-cup) servings PREP TIME: 10 minutes COOK TIME: 18 to 20 minutes

1 cup toasted
  buckwheat groats
1¾ cups water
1 tablespoon
  unsalted
  butter or oil
2 tablespoons
  water, breast
  milk, or formula
  (optional)
¾ cup plain full-fat
  Greek yogurt
½ cup Roasted
  Pear and Date
  Puree (page 66;
  optional)

Buckwheat is a popular grain around the world, but it doesn't get the recognition it deserves here in the United States. Buckwheat is gluten-free (for those who need to avoid gluten, see page 6) and a natural source of iron, protein, and fiber.

1. Using a colander, rinse and drain the buckwheat well.

2. In a medium saucepan, combine the buckwheat, water, and butter or oil. Bring to a boil, then cover tightly and simmer over low heat for 18 to 20 minutes.

3. If you prefer a smoother texture, allow to cool for 10 minutes.

4. Place the buckwheat in a blender or food processor and add the water, breast milk, or formula, 2 tablespoons at a time, while blending until smooth.

5. To serve, top each serving with 1 tablespoon of the yogurt. If desired, add a dollop of the sweet pear and date puree to increase the nutrition and depth of flavor.

TEXTURE TIP: Introducing your baby to new textures, like the cooked buckwheat, can help them master more complex ways of moving their oral muscles. This increases texture exposure, helping to prevent those "picky" tendencies that may pop up later, while also getting those muscles ready for speech!

BAKED SALMON AND SWEET POTATO PUREE

GLUTEN-FREE **NUT-FREE**

YIELD: 16 (2-ounce/¼-cup) servings **PREP TIME:** 10 minutes, plus 1 hour to cool
COOK TIME: 1 hour 15 minutes

Nonstick cooking
  spray (optional)
2 wild-caught
  salmon fillets
  (5 to 7 ounces
  each), either fresh
  or frozen and
  defrosted
4 medium sweet
  potatoes
1 garlic clove, diced
½ teaspoon
  onion powder
1 teaspoon unsalted
  butter, melted
½ cup low- or
  no-sodium
  vegetable broth
  (or breast milk,
  formula, or cow's
  milk/non-dairy
  alternative)

Fish can provide so many health benefits, such as
brain-boosting fat and immune-supporting vitamin D, so
helping your baby get familiar with it now will go a long way
toward food acceptance in the future.

1. Preheat the oven to 400°F. Line a baking sheet with parchment
   paper or use aluminum foil and coat it with cooking spray.

2. Wash the sweet potatoes, then poke each 5 to 7 times with a
   fork. Place on the baking sheet and bake for 1 hour. Remove
   and let cool, about 20 minutes.

3. Again, line the baking sheet with parchment paper or
   aluminum foil and coat the foil with cooking spray. Lay the
   salmon fillets skin side down on the baking sheet.

4. Combine the garlic, onion powder, and butter in a small
   bowl. Brush onto the salmon, then bake for 15 minutes, or to
   an internal temperature of 145°F.

5. Cool the salmon in the refrigerator for 1 hour. If desired,
   remove the skin (see Nutrition Tip), then cut the salmon into
   medium pieces.

6. Scoop out the sweet potato flesh and place it in a
   high-powered blender or food processor. Add the salmon
   and broth and blend until the desired consistency is reached.

NUTRITION TIP: Much of the delicious, beneficial fat in the salmon is
in the skin..

POTATO, CARROT, AND SWEET CORN PUREE

GLUTEN-FREE NUT-FREE VEGETARIAN

YIELD: 16 (2-ounce/¼-cup) servings **PREP TIME:** 10 minutes, plus 15 to 20 minutes to cool
COOK TIME: 25 minutes

1 tablespoon
  unsalted butter
½ medium onion,
  chopped
2 medium carrots,
  chopped
2 medium waxy
  potatoes, peeled
  and chopped
1 cup fresh, canned,
  or thawed frozen
  corn kernel (see
  Cooking tip)
¾ cup no- or
  low-sodium
  vegetable broth

White potatoes provide so many sources of delicious nutrition, including potassium, vitamin C, magnesium, phosphorus, calcium, iron, and zinc! Corn provides lutein and zeaxanthin, two phytochemicals that promote healthy vision. Along with the soluble fiber that helps promote a healthy gut, corn also has B vitamins, iron, protein, and potassium.

1. Heat a medium saucepan over medium heat. Add the butter and let it melt. As it begins to brown, add the onion and sauté for about 1 minute, until fragrant.

2. Add the carrots and sauté for an additional 5 minutes, until soft.

3. Add the potatoes and the broth, and cook for 12 to 15 minutes, until the potatoes are tender when poked with a fork.

4. If using fresh corn, add it to the pot now and cook for another 3 to 5 minutes.

5. Remove the saucepan from the heat and let the mixture cool for 15 to 20 minutes.

6. Using a slotted spoon, transfer the onion, carrots, potatoes, and corn to a blender or food processor. If using thawed or canned corn, add that now. Blend to the desired consistency, adding some of the cooking liquid, 1 tablespoon at a time, as needed. If desired, push the mixture through a sieve for a creamier puree.

COOKING TIP: While many of us have heard that canning vegetables renders them devoid of nutrition, that's not actually true. The canning process does slightly reduce the amount of vitamin C and certain B vitamins, but not in a meaningful way. Both vitamins C and B are found in many foods, so the slight reduction when using canned produce isn't a serious problem. Choose cans that are BPA-free and free of dents.

MANGO, APPLE, AND SPINACH PUREE

DAIRY-FREE   GLUTEN-FREE   NUT-FREE   VEGAN

YIELD: 12 (2-ounce/¼-cup) servings   **PREP TIME:** 10 minutes, plus 10 minutes to cool
COOK TIME: 20 to 25 minutes

Nonstick cooking
  spray (optional)
1 medium mango,
  cut into chunks
2 apples (any
  variety), peeled,
  cored, and
  chopped
3 cups (packed)
  baby spinach

I tell my kids all the time that it's important to experience all five flavors—sweet, salty, bitter, sour, and umami (savory-delicious)—each day. A meal that includes multiple flavors is more satisfying. This recipe incorporates three of those flavors and goes a long way toward encouraging food enjoyment! While we don't give much added salt to little ones, they can pick up subtle natural flavors with their super-delicate taste buds.

1. Preheat the oven to 350°F. Line a baking sheet with parchment paper or use aluminum foil and lightly coat it with cooking spray.

2. Arrange the fruit on the baking sheet in a single layer. Bake for 20 to 25 minutes, or until tender.

3. Allow to cool for 10 minutes.

4. Add the fruit to a blender or food processor and blend to the desired consistency, adding the spinach 1 cup at a time and fully incorporating each cup before adding the next one.

TEXTURE TIP: If you are ready for a chunkier consistency, use a potato masher instead of a blender to mash the apples and mango. Save the spinach for another recipe!

PLANTAIN, CARROT, AND CHICKEN PUREE

DAIRY-FREE **GLUTEN-FREE** **NUT-FREE**

YIELD: 16 (2-ounce/¼-cup) servings **PREP TIME:** 10 minutes, plus 20 minutes to cool
COOK TIME: 25 minutes

1 ripe plantain (see
    Cooking tip)
1½ teaspoons
    olive oil or
    unsalted butter
½ small onion,
    chopped
2 medium carrots,
    chopped
1 cup no- or
    low-sodium
    chicken or
    vegetable broth
1 (5- to 6-ounce)
    skinless, boneless
    chicken breast
    or equivalent
    in boneless
    thighs, chopped

Meat is a wonderful first food. It's not often considered because it doesn't blend easily, and it can taste dry to new eaters. By combining chicken with starchy plantains and carrots, though, you can provide your baby with a delicious and nutritious meal that's also creamy.

1. Cut off the top and bottom of the plantain, then cut the rest of the fruit in half crosswise. Remove the peel.

2. Heat the oil or butter in a medium saucepan over medium heat. Add the onion and sauté until soft, 2 to 3 minutes.

3. Add the carrots and plantain, then pour in the broth and bring to a boil. Reduce the heat, cover, and cook for 10 minutes.

4. Add the chicken and continue to cook for 10 minutes more, until the chicken is cooked through and the carrots and plantain are soft.

5. Remove from the heat and allow to cool for about 20 minutes.

6. Using a slotted spoon, transfer the solid ingredients to a blender or food processor and blend until smooth, adding a little reserved cooking liquid as needed for a smooth puree.

COOKING TIP: Choose a plantain that is firm to the touch and relatively free of spots. A ripe plantain will be yellow with slightly green ends; a plantain that's too ripe will be almost black and is too soft for this preparation.

BLUEBERRY AND CHICKPEA PUREE

30 MINUTES OR LESS | **DAIRY-FREE** | **GLUTEN-FREE** | **NUT-FREE** | **VEGAN**

YIELD: 8 (2-ounce/¼-cup) servings **PREP TIME:** 5 minutes

1 cup fresh or
frozen blueberries

1 cup canned
low-sodium or
home-cooked
chickpeas, rinsed
and drained (see
Cooking Tip)

¼ cup water

While varieties of hummus are relatively new in the Western Hemisphere, people in North Africa and the Middle East have counted chickpeas among their dietary staples for thousands of years. Chickpeas, also called garbanzo beans, are high in folate, fiber, protein, and many micronutrients. Their fun shape and creamy texture make them a great food to include in your baby's regular meal rotation.

Place the blueberries and chickpeas in a blender or food processor. Blend until smooth, adding the water 1 tablespoon at a time, to the desired consistency.

COOKING TIP: If you're reconstituting dried chickpeas, the easiest method is to put them in the slow cooker, cover with water, and cook on high for 3 hours.

BANANA AND PEANUT BUTTER PUREE

30 MINUTES OR LESS | GLUTEN-FREE | VEGETARIAN

YIELD: 4 (2-ounce/¼-cup) servings PREP TIME: 5 minutes

1 firm, ripe banana

2 tablespoons natural peanut butter

¼ cup cow's milk or non-dairy alternative, as needed

From current research, we know that it's best to introduce your baby early on to allergenic foods such as peanut butter as a way to prevent allergies. If peanut butter isn't a good option for your family, you can substitute any other seed or nut butter in this recipe.

1. Peel the banana and place it in a blender or food processor.

2. Add the peanut butter and milk and blend to the desired consistency.

TEXTURE TIP: The actual amount of milk you'll use will depend on the size and ripeness of the banana. Add just enough to obtain the desired texture.

ADDITION TIP: Add a pinch of ground cinnamon to increase the flavor and fun!

MEAL TIP: Serve with yogurt or oatmeal for a delicious breakfast.

MASHED POTATOES

`30 MINUTES OR LESS` `GLUTEN-FREE` `NUT-FREE` `VEGETARIAN`

YIELD: 4 (2-ounce/¼-cup) servings **PREP TIME:** 10 minutes **COOK TIME:** 15 minutes

8 cups water
1 tablespoon kosher salt
1 pound waxy potatoes (such as Yukon Gold), peeled and quartered
1 tablespoon unsalted butter
½ cup cow's milk or non-dairy alternative

This recipe will stick around long after your baby is out of diapers. Mashed potatoes are a comforting, creamy side dish that pairs well with salmon, meats, or an all-veggie extravaganza. You'll notice that the water here is salted. Most of this salt will go down the drain after the potatoes cook, which makes this recipe safe for your baby.

1. In a large pot, bring the water and salt to a boil.

2. Add the potatoes and cook just until tender, about 15 minutes. Test with a knife.

3. Transfer the boiled potatoes to a blender or food processor. Add the butter and milk, and blend until smooth. Alternatively, drain the potatoes and return them to the pot; add the butter and milk, and use either a potato masher or an immersion blender to puree your potatoes.

TEXTURE TIP: As your baby grows and is able to tolerate more salt, you can add salt and pepper to taste. Experiment with different textures as your baby grows—creamy mashed potatoes are a different experience from chunkier ones.

TOFU AND SWEET POTATO MASH

30 MINUTES OR LESS | **GLUTEN-FREE** | **NUT-FREE** | **VEGETARIAN**

YIELD: 3 (2-ounce/¼-cup) servings **PREP TIME:** 5 minutes, plus 10 minutes to cool
COOK TIME: 15 minutes

1 medium sweet
potato, peeled
and chopped
2 tablespoons
silken tofu
¼ cup cow's milk,
breast milk,
formula, or
non-dairy milk

Tofu is a fantastic source of protein, calcium, and iron—
all important nutrients for a growing child. Tofu is widely
available, inexpensive, and so versatile.

1. Using a stovetop steamer insert or a microwave, steam the
   sweet potato until tender, about 15 minutes for stovetop and
   5 minutes for microwave. Allow to cool for about 10 minutes.

2. Place the sweet potato in a blender or food processor. Add
   the tofu, and blend to the desired consistency, adding
   the milk, breast milk, or formula, 1 tablespoon at a time,
   as needed.

STORAGE TIP: Did you know that you can freeze tofu? Simply cut
it into cubes, fast-freeze it on a baking sheet for 3 to 4 hours, then
transfer it to a freezer-safe container for up to 3 months.

OVERNIGHT CHIA PUDDING

GLUTEN-FREE **NUT-FREE** **VEGETARIAN**

YIELD: 5 (2-ounce/¼-cup) servings **PREP TIME:** 5 minutes, plus overnight to thicken

4 tablespoons
white or black
chia seeds

1 cup cow's milk
or non-dairy
alternative

3 to 3½ tablespoons
sweet puree
of choice (see
Addition Tip)

Growing chia seeds was a popular activity in the 1980s, when the Chia Pet graced so many kitchen windows. Now, chia seeds have gained popularity as a nutritious addition to oatmeal and baked goods, or as the basis for chia pudding. This puree has quite a bit of texture, so it's a great new food to expose to your baby.

1. In a mason jar or other lidded container, combine the chia seeds and milk. Let the mixture sit overnight in the refrigerator. The pudding will thicken somewhat.

2. When you're ready to serve the pudding, stir it well, then pour into your baby's dish. Add up to 2 teaspoons of the sweet puree per serving for flavoring.

ADDITION TIP: This pudding is bland, so adding a bit of sweet puree heightens the enjoyment. Try Roasted Banana Puree (page 25), Stone Fruit Slow Cooker Puree (page 50), or Papaya Puree (page 39).

TEXTURE TIP: If you prefer a smoother texture, blend the ingredients in a high-powered blender before refrigerating it overnight.

PEACH, RASPBERRY, AND QUINOA PUREE

GLUTEN-FREE NUT-FREE VEGETARIAN

YIELD: 16 (2-ounce/¼-cup) servings **PREP TIME:** 10 minutes, plus 10 minutes to rest
COOK TIME: 15 minutes

½ cup white quinoa

1 cup water

3 ripe peaches, peeled and pitted, or 1 (15-ounce) package frozen peaches, thawed

1 cup fresh or frozen raspberries

½ cup cow's milk or non-dairy alternative

Quinoa, pronounced KEEN-wah, is considered a pseudo-cereal grain but is actually a seed. Its recent popularity can be attributed to its versatility, taste, and texture. Quinoa can be part of a nutritious breakfast when served cold with yogurt and berries, or it can be a warm and savory side dish when prepared with broth, veggies, and seasonings. This recipe introduces your new eater to white quinoa, which has a milder taste and softer texture.

1. In a medium saucepan, cook the quinoa according to package instructions, usually 15 minutes to cook and 10 minutes to rest.

2. Place the peaches and raspberries in a blender or food processor and blend, adding the milk, 1 tablespoon at a time, to the desired consistency.

3. Fluff the quinoa, then gently mix in the puree. (If a smoother texture is desired, add the quinoa to the blender or food processor along with the fruit and milk.)

TEXTURE TIP: It's essential to begin exposing your baby to different textures as they grow. More complex textures will work your baby's oral muscles, preparing them for language!

ROASTED PEAR AND DATE PUREE

DAIRY-FREE GLUTEN-FREE NUT-FREE VEGAN

YIELD: 10 (2-ounce/¼ cup) servings **PREP TIME:** 10 minutes **COOK TIME:** 30 minutes

Nonstick cooking
  spray (optional)
3 medium pears,
  peeled, cored,
  and sliced
¼ teaspoon ground
  cinnamon
5 Medjool dates,
  pitted
½ cup hot water

There is something decadent about roasted pears—and dates, too! This sumptuous puree will be wonderful for your baby when served with yogurt or oatmeal. If you are looking for a treat for yourself, consider spreading this puree on crostini smeared with goat cheese and maybe a drizzle of honey.

1. Preheat the oven to 425°F. Line a baking sheet with parchment paper or use aluminum foil and coat it lightly with cooking spray.

2. Lay the pear slices on the baking sheet in a single layer. Lightly sprinkle the cinnamon over the pears. Bake for 30 minutes, or until soft. Let cool.

3. Meanwhile, cover the dates with the hot water and let soak for 10 minutes (or longer). Drain and reserve the soaking liquid.

4. Place the roasted pears and the dates in a blender or food processor and blend to the desired consistency, adding some of the soaking liquid, 1 tablespoon at a time, as needed.

SUBSTITUTION TIP: Medjool dates are large, dark, and deliciously squishy. You can use other date varieties, but as they may be smaller, you may have to increase the amount. For example, Deglet Noor dates are smaller and have less flesh, with a larger pit, so you'll need to double the number of dates used.

BUTTERNUT SQUASH, CHERRY, AND MILLET PUREE

GLUTEN-FREE **NUT-FREE** **VEGETARIAN**

YIELD: 16 (2-ounce/¼-cup) servings **PREP TIME:** 10 minutes, plus 20 minutes to rest
COOK TIME: 35 minutes

½ cup millet

1 cup water

Scant 2 cups Roasted Butternut Squash Puree (page 29)

1 cup fresh or frozen sweet cherries, pitted

¼ cup cow's milk or non-dairy alternative (optional)

This recipe builds on a puree of butternut squash to make a sweet, tart, and textured meal for your growing baby. Cherries are full of antioxidants to support the immune system. Millet supports intestinal health and promotes regular bowel movements.

1. In a small saucepan, toast the millet over medium heat for 4 to 5 minutes, until it just begins to brown.

2. Add the water and bring to a boil. Reduce the heat to low, cover, and simmer for 30 minutes. Remove the saucepan from the heat and let rest, covered, for another 20 minutes.

3. Place the millet, squash puree, and cherries in a blender or food processor and blend to the desired consistency, adding the milk, 1 tablespoon at a time, as desired for smoothness.

NUTRITION TIP: Millet is actually a grass, native to Asia and Africa. There is evidence that we have been consuming it for the past 7,000 years! Millet is high in protein, fiber, and several of the B vitamins.

SPINACH AND APPLE PUREE

DAIRY-FREE GLUTEN-FREE NUT-FREE VEGAN

YIELD: 16 (2-ounce/¼-cup) servings **PREP TIME:** 5 minutes, plus 15 minutes to cool
COOK TIME: 15 minutes

6 apples (any
  variety), peeled,
  cored, and
  chopped
2 cups (packed)
  baby spinach,
  or ⅔ cup frozen
  chopped spinach
½ teaspoon ground
  cinnamon

Spinach and apple pair so nicely. The subtle, bitter flavors of the spinach are offset by the sweetness of the apple. Spinach is a good source of iron, which is even more available when the spinach is cooked. Apples are a wonderful source of soluble fiber, essential for keeping tummies happy.

1. Using a stovetop steamer insert or a microwave, steam the apples for 15 minutes, until soft.

2. Remove the steamer from the heat, add the spinach, and let sit, covered, for 2 more minutes, then cool completely.

3. Drain the spinach and apples, reserving 2 tablespoons of the cooking liquid.

4. Place the apples, spinach, and cinnamon in a blender or food processor and blend to the desired consistency, adding some of the reserved cooking liquid, 1 tablespoon at a time, as needed.

NUTRITION TIP: Did you know that spinach contains more potassium than bananas? Potassium is necessary for cell function, regulating heartbeat, ensuring optimal function of muscles and nerves, and synthesizing protein and metabolizing carbohydrates.

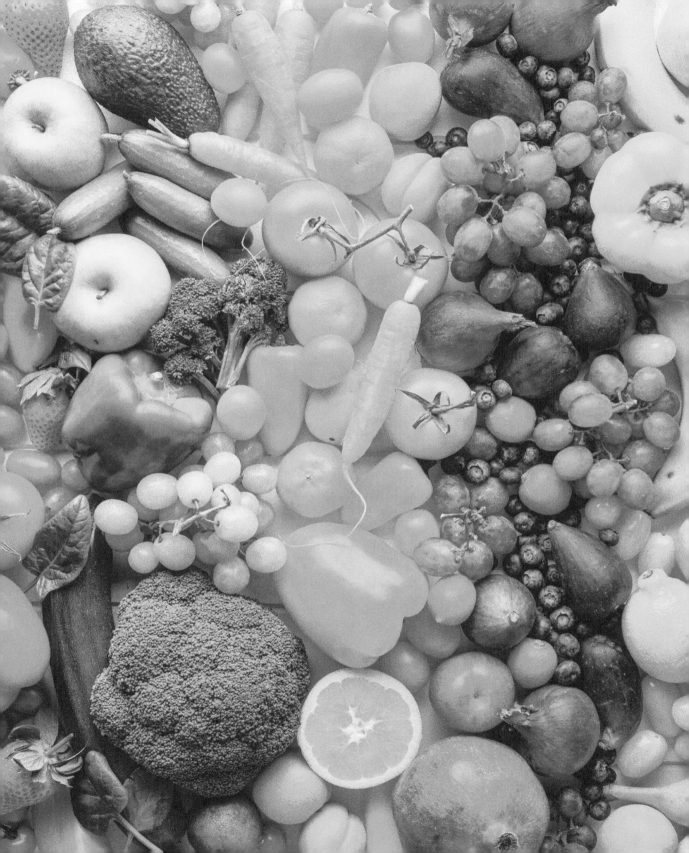

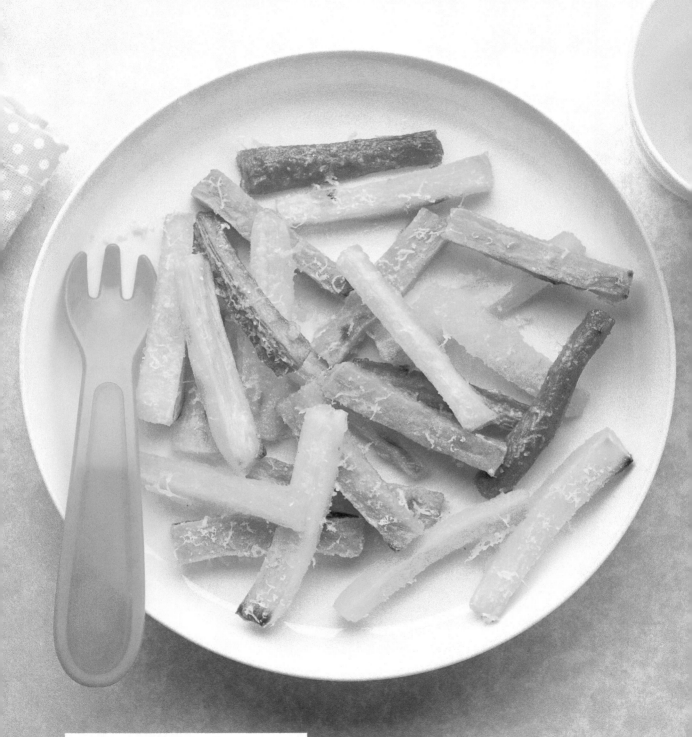

MIXED ROOT-VEGGIE FRIES PAGE 88

4

9 TO 12 MONTHS

SMOOTHIES AND SOFT FINGER FOODS

OPTIMAL NUTRITION

Until this point, you may have been heavily involved in feeding your little one—helping them use their spoon, watching carefully for those wide-open eyes and that interested forward lean, mouth open and waiting for the deliciousness yet to come. Now is the time to put your baby in the driver's seat (but not literally—you still have about 16 years for that!). It's finger-food time! To keep this period safe and enjoyable, be aware of choking hazards (see page 9).

This chapter explores new tastes and textures. New experiences represent new exposure to a variety of nutrients. Each color is a world of its own, providing unique health benefits. By creating a rainbow on your plate—over the course of a day, not at each meal—you can provide the optimal nutrition for your growing little one.

MAINTAINING BREAST MILK OR FORMULA

Breast milk or formula still represents your baby's primary nutrition, but this is about to change. At 9 to 12 months, you provide your baby with liquid nutrition prior to a solid-food meal (including any purees), but you can also begin to space out the meals to allow for a bit of an appetite to develop. Solid foods should not be given more than about 45 minutes after the breast or bottle, to avoid the risk of interfering with your baby's appetite for the next liquid meal.

IMPORTANT NUTRIENTS

Breast milk or formula remains your baby's primary source of nutrition, so the only nutrients that must be derived from solid food or supplements are still iron, zinc, and vitamin D. After the 12-month mark, your baby will be dependent on solid food for nutrition. Breast milk will remain a nutritious and comforting option, but formula can be replaced with cow's milk or a non-dairy alternative. This is discussed more in chapter 5.

FOODS TO EMBRACE

This time is a golden opportunity. Your baby loves and trusts you implicitly. Most foods you present to your baby are accepted with a smile, a giggle, or a scream of delight. Food has been an adventure. In the next chapter, I discuss how to handle the shift, as your baby may begin to be wary of new food experiences. But at this moment, present your baby with a variety of colors, flavors, and textures. Make everything familiar. Feed with joy, and your baby will associate the table atmosphere with comfort and love.

FOODS TO WAIT ON

Honey and salt remain on the list of foods to avoid. Your baby's immune system is getting stronger and the kidneys are developing. At 12 months, honey and salt will no longer be much of an issue. Continue to mind the choking hazards until age 4 (see page 9).

UNDERSTANDING BABY'S DEVELOPMENT

Feeding is more than just providing nutrition; it is inextricably linked to various fine and gross motor skills. In fact, it is at the table where you first might notice a slight delay or advancement in physical development. So, it's essential to keep in mind that all developmental milestones occur within a range. If you have any concerns about your baby's physical development, please speak with your doctor.

PALMAR AND PINCER GRASP

The *palmar* grasp is the grasp that occurs when you stimulate a child's palm and they grab on with their full fist. This is how they have been interacting with objects up to this point. At 9 months, the child likely has a defined *pincer* grasp, which is the coordination of the index finger and thumb. It's common to encourage a child to develop this skill by providing cereals like Cheerios. Watch their wonder as they grasp the cereal between their two fingers.

INTRODUCING SIPPY CUPS

Stick with sippy cups that resemble big kid cups; this will ease the transition to an open cup later. A soft-tipped straw cup, for example, is easy on baby's teeth and looks a lot like the cup your baby might see you enjoying after hitting the

Starbucks drive-through. In fact, Starbucks has a kid-size water cup! Enjoying a beverage together, using similar cups, can really help grow your child's interest. Start this process sooner rather than later, since the American Academy of Pediatrics recommends leaving behind the baby bottle by 18 months.

NEW TOOLS AND UTENSILS

As your child becomes more confident in their gripping and grabbing skills, it is even more important to model good eating behavior at the table. No, I'm not talking about sitting politely with a cloth napkin on the lap. I'm talking about demonstrating how to use a fork, how to drink from an open or straw cup, and how to enjoy time at the table. Consider upgrading your child's fork and spoon to a set that more closely resembles yours, remembering that your baby will continue to use child-size utensils until at least 2 years old. Select cups that feature a beloved character or favorite color. Interact with your child by "toasting" or crunching at the same time. Model your food enjoyment; the rest will follow.

TYPICAL MEALS AND SCHEDULE

There isn't a single schedule that works for everyone. On the facing page is a sample schedule, offered to illustrate the timing expected between meals and snacks. A meal should consist of two or three different items, and a snack should generally include two food items. Each meal or snack should contain fat, protein, and carbohydrates in order to be filling and satisfying. Your child's stomach is the same size as their fist, a fact that remains true through adulthood. They may eat more than this volume, but in case you get concerned that they are not eating enough, that visual will help put you at ease.

Sample Meal Schedule

6:00 A.M.	Wake and feed (breast milk or formula)
7:45 A.M.	Solid food breakfast
8:00 A.M.	Morning nap (45 to 60 minutes or more)
9:00 A.M.	Wake and feed (breast milk or formula)
9:45 A.M.	Snack 1
12:00 P.M.	Nap (1½ to 2 hours or more)
2:00 P.M.	Wake and feed (breast milk or formula)
2:45 P.M.	Snack 2
5:00 P.M.	Solid food dinner
5:30 P.M.	Begin bedtime routine
6:00 P.M.	Breast milk or formula, then to bed

COMMON CHALLENGES

Here are some common challenges at this age.

YOUR CHILD ISN'T EATING ENOUGH OR IS EATING TOO MUCH.

Parents have an idea about how much their children *should* be eating, right? The truth is that our job is to encourage our children to listen to their own bodies for signals of hunger and fullness. If food is presented in a pressure-free and joyful way, your child will likely eat exactly the amount that fills them up—no more and no less. That may sometimes mean that they choose to skip a meal or that they eat the amount you would expect an adult to consume. Provide the amount of food the child requests; they will be communicating with screaming, laughter, or signing at this point. Sit with your child the same way as you would sit with a guest at your table, enjoying a pleasant moment together.

YOUR CHILD IS POCKETING FOOD.

If your child is pocketing food, stuffing the mouth and keeping food in the space between the cheeks and gums, it could be a sign that your child is eating too quickly before mastering all the oral-motor skills required for eating. If it becomes a persistent concern, you may find confidence by touching base with a feeding specialist. Here are some tips:

1. Help your baby slow down by giving them one or two pieces of food at a time.

2. Offer frequent sips of water.

3. Use cookie cutters or a fun food cutter to create bite-size pieces.

4. Talk to each other at the table, and not just about chewing food.

5. Avoid distractions at the table, such as TV or other screens. These can contribute to less-than-mindful eating.

6. Consider whether you're pressuring your child to eat, then take a step back and give your child some space to explore their food.

ORANGE DREAMSICLE SMOOTHIE

30 MINUTES OR LESS | **GLUTEN-FREE** | **NUT-FREE** | **VEGETARIAN**

YIELD: 4 (4-ounce/½-cup) servings **PREP TIME:** 5 minutes

½ cup plain full-fat Greek yogurt

1 cup cow's milk or non-dairy alternative

1 medium banana, frozen

1 orange or 2 clementines, peeled and segmented

½ teaspoon no-alcohol vanilla extract

I have a fond memory of eating Creamsicles in my parents' bed way past my bedtime. The flavor is such a comforting memory for me.

1. Place the yogurt, milk, banana, and orange in a blender or food processor.

2. Add the vanilla and then blend until smooth, about 2 minutes.

NUTRITION TIP: While this smoothie is full of nutrition, it might not be the best option for a baby who is having a bit of constipation. If your baby hasn't had a bowel movement in more than a day, try the Sweet Berry Constipation Smoothie (page 78) instead.

MAKE-AHEAD TIP: You can prep these smoothies ahead of time by blending everything except for the frozen banana, then storing in the fridge for 2 to 3 days. When you're ready to serve, just add the frozen banana and blend. If you've got some leftovers, consider making ice pops!

SWEET BERRY CONSTIPATION SMOOTHIE

30 MINUTES OR LESS | **GLUTEN-FREE** | **NUT-FREE** | **VEGETARIAN**

YIELD: 12 (2-ounce/¼-cup) servings **PREP TIME:** 5 minutes

½ cup pure, unsweetened apple juice

2 prunes, pitted

4 Medjool dates, pitted

½ cup plain whole-fat kefir or non-dairy alternative

½ tablespoon hulled hemp hearts

1 tablespoon chia seeds

1 cup fresh or frozen blueberries

6 to 8 fresh strawberries, hulled

1 tablespoon coconut oil, melted

½ to 1 teaspoon ground cinnamon

3 or 4 ice cubes (optional)

"Dirty diapers daily!" Say it with me! This amazing recipe will really get things moving, for both the littles and the adults. This recipe comes courtesy of Feeding Littles, a great online resource for child nutrition. It's intended to be used in small doses, almost medicinally rather than as a snack. Start with a 2-ounce (¼ cup) serving for a child 6 to 12 months old and increase to 4 ounces (½ cup) for a child over 12 months old. Serve two to three times per day until constipation is resolved.

1. Pour the apple juice into a high-powered blender.

2. Add the prunes, dates, kefir, hemp hearts, chia seeds, blueberries, strawberries, coconut oil, cinnamon, and ice (if using).

3. Blend for 30 seconds, or until the hemp hearts are completely blended and the mixture is smooth.

NUTRITION TIP: Kefir is a fermented milk drink that originated in Eastern Europe. Much like yogurt, it is full of beneficial bacteria to support gut health and the immune system. Compared to yogurt, kefir generally has a much higher concentration and variety of good bacteria.

MAKE-AHEAD TIP: You can prep these smoothies ahead of time by blending everything except for the frozen berries and ice cubes, then storing in the fridge for 2 to 3 days. When you're ready to serve, just add the frozen berries and ice cubes and blend. If you've got some leftovers, consider making ice pops!

BERRY AND SPINACH SMOOTHIE

30 MINUTES OR LESS | GLUTEN-FREE | NUT-FREE | VEGETARIAN

YIELD: 6 (4-ounce/½-cup) servings **PREP TIME:** 5 minutes

1 cup plain full-fat
Greek yogurt
or non-dairy
alternative

2 cups
frozen berries

1 orange or
2 clementines,
peeled and
segmented

¼ cup (packed)
trimmed
fresh spinach

7 or 8 fresh
strawberries,
hulled

Maybe I'm not supposed to be biased, but this is my favorite smoothie. I just love the sweet-tartness of the berries and the happy energy boost that comes from fresh spinach. These aspects are brought together beautifully with creamy yogurt to provide a satisfying and refreshing smoothie that pairs well with any meal or snack.

1. Place the yogurt in a blender or food processor.

2. Add the berries, orange segments, spinach, and strawberries, and blend until smooth, about 3 minutes.

MAKE-AHEAD TIP: You can prep these smoothies ahead of time by blending everything except the frozen berries, then storing in the refrigerator for 2 to 3 days. When you're ready to serve, just add the frozen berries and blend. If you've got some leftovers, consider making ice pops!

CHOCOLATE-DATE SMOOTHIE

30 MINUTES OR LESS | **GLUTEN-FREE** | **VEGETARIAN**

YIELD: 2 (4-ounce/½-cup) servings **PREP TIME:** 5 minutes

¾ cup cow's milk or non-dairy alternative

¼ cup whole hazelnuts (with or without skin), soaked overnight and drained

1 tablespoon unsweetened cocoa powder

3 or 4 Medjool dates, pitted

It's so much fun to share our favorite flavors with our kids. This smoothie tastes just like Nutella! While your little one might be too young to enjoy the glory that is a Nutella and banana crepe, you can start them on this delicious treat. Note: The hazelnuts need to be soaked overnight.

1. Pour the milk into a blender or food processor.

2. Add the hazelnuts, cocoa, and dates, and blend until smooth, 3 to 4 minutes.

NUTRITION TIP: For a nutrition boost, add 1 tablespoon of chia seeds to the blender. If you don't have hazelnuts, you can use ¼ cup nut butter of your choice.

MAKE-AHEAD TIP: You can prep these smoothies ahead of time by blending everything except the frozen berries, then storing in the fridge for 2 to 3 days. If you've got some leftovers, consider making ice pops!

TROPICAL MANGO SMOOTHIE

30 MINUTES OR LESS | GLUTEN-FREE | NUT-FREE | VEGETARIAN

YIELD: 6 (4-ounce/½-cup) servings **PREP TIME:** 5 minutes

½ cup cow's milk
or non-dairy
alternative

½ cup plain full-fat
Greek yogurt
or non-dairy
alternative

2 ripe mangos,
chopped, or
2 cups frozen
mango cubes

1 medium banana,
peeled, chopped,
and frozen, or
1 fresh banana
if using frozen
mango

This wonderful, creamy smoothie is a vacation in a cup. While you can use either frozen bananas or frozen mango, using both will result in a smoothie that refuses to blend. Pick one frozen and the other fresh, or simply allow one to fully thaw prior to blending.

1. Pour the milk into a blender or food processor and add the yogurt.

2. Add the mango and banana, and blend until completely smooth.

NUTRITION TIP: There are hundreds of types of mangos, but they all are high in vitamin C, folate, and vitamin B_6. And that's not all: mangos are also creamy and dreamy to eat.

MAKE-AHEAD TIP: You can prep these smoothies ahead of time by blending everything except for the frozen fruit, then storing in the fridge for 2 to 3 days. When you're ready to serve, just add the frozen fruit and blend. If you've got some leftovers, consider making ice pops!

AVOCADO FOUR WAYS

30 MINUTES OR LESS **GLUTEN-FREE** **NUT-FREE** **VEGETARIAN**

The avocado is a fascinating plant. Botanically, it's a fruit but culinarily, it's a vegetable. And nutritionally, it's an oil! Avocado is mild-tasting with a creamy texture, so it's wonderful for adding to pureed foods, using as a sandwich spread, or making guacamole. It is a great first food and a nice addition to so many meals throughout one's life.

AVOCADO WEDGES

YIELD: 4 or 5 slices PREP TIME: 5 minutes

½ Hass avocado

1. Place the half without the pit flat side down on a cutting board and slice directly through the flesh and skin.

2. Peel off half the skin, leaving the skin on the lower half of each avocado slice for gripping purposes.

3. Serve the slices to your baby and watch them enjoy being in control of their own bite!

AVOCADO TOAST

YIELD: 4 strips PREP TIME: 1 minute
COOK TIME: 4 minutes

1 slice whole wheat bread
¼ section of Hass avocado

1. Toast the bread in a toaster or under the broiler until golden brown.

2. Scoop the avocado flesh out of the skin and spread on the bread.

3. Slice the bread into 4 strips and serve!

SIMPLE GUACAMOLE

YIELD: 6 (2-ounce/¼ cup) servings
PREP TIME: 5 minutes

2 Hass avocados
1 garlic clove, diced
Juice of 1 lime

1. Scoop the flesh out of the avocados into a small bowl. Reserve one of the pits.

2. Using a fork, smash the avocado to the desired consistency, keeping it a little chunky.

3. Add the garlic and lime juice, and stir to incorporate.

STORAGE TIP: Store any leftover guacamole in the bowl in the refrigerator with the pit in the center and covered tightly in plastic wrap with the wrap touching the surface to prevent browning. It will keep for about 3 days.

AVOCADO EGG SALAD

YIELD: 3 (4-ounce/½-cup) servings
PREP TIME: 5 minutes

½ Hass avocado
2 hard-boiled eggs, peeled
2 tablespoons cooked quinoa

1. Using a potato masher or a fork, mash the avocado and eggs together in a small bowl.

2. Mix in the quinoa and serve.

NUTRITION TIP: Fat is an essential part of the human diet. Not only does it support a baby's brain development, but as a child grows it can also help with mood regulation. Fat aids with the absorption of vitamins A, D, E, and K, and it also helps the body produce important hormones.

VERY VEGGIE PATTIES

30 MINUTES OR LESS | DAIRY-FREE | GLUTEN-FREE | NUT-FREE | ONE PAN | VEGAN

YIELD: 10 small patties **PREP TIME:** 15 minutes **COOK TIME:** 5 to 8 minutes

1 (15-ounce) can low-sodium chickpeas or black beans

1 cup gluten-free old-fashioned rolled oats

¼ cup ground flax seeds

1 cup shredded carrots (about 2 medium)

½ cup frozen peas

1 tablespoon minced garlic

½ cup chopped onion

2 teaspoons ground cumin (optional)

Nonstick cooking spray (optional)

These veggie burgers are the perfect way to boost the number of vegetables in your meal plan. Once you get the hang of the cooking method, you'll be able to incorporate leftover veggies to create a deliciously repurposed meal. While you can make these on the stovetop or an electric griddle, it's easiest in a panini press or a countertop electric grill.

1. Combine the chickpeas, oats, flax seeds, carrots, peas, garlic, onion, and cumin (if using) in a large bowl.

2. Using a potato masher, mash the ingredients together until well blended.

3. Form 10 patties, about ⅓ cup each, by spooning out portions of the mixture and rolling them into balls, then flattening them into patties.

4. Either sauté the patties in a medium skillet coated with non-stick cooking spray over high heat for 3 to 4 minutes on each side or grill in a panini press until golden, 5 to 6 minutes.

NUTRITION TIP: Chickpeas are amazingly versatile and work well also in salads or for making hummus. They're naturally high in folate, fiber, and protein.

QUICK AND DELICIOUS EGG MUFFINS

GLUTEN-FREE **NUT-FREE** **ONE PAN** **VEGETARIAN**

YIELD: 12 muffins **PREP TIME:** 10 minutes, plus 10 minutes to cool **COOK TIME:** 20 minutes

Nonstick cooking
  spray (optional)
12 large eggs
2 tablespoons finely
  chopped onion
¼ cup roughly
  chopped
  fresh spinach
8 grape or cherry
  tomatoes, cut
  into halves
¼ cup shredded
  mozzarella

These super simple egg muffins are great for snacks or meals. They freeze and reheat well, and they travel well, too! This is the limitless toddler meal! You can make the basic mixture, then add different veggies to each muffin for variety, or you can make confetti egg muffins by including colorful veggies in each.

1. Preheat the oven to 350°F. Lightly spray a 12-cup muffin tin with cooking spray or line with muffin liners.

2. In a large bowl, whisk together the eggs and onion.

3. Mix in the spinach, cherry tomatoes, and cheese.

4. Distribute the batter evenly among the muffin cups and bake the muffins for 20 minutes, until puffed and rounded on top.

5. Cool for 10 minutes before releasing from the tin.

STORAGE TIP: To freeze the muffins, wrap each cooled muffin in plastic wrap and freeze for up to 2 months. To reheat, simply unwrap and microwave in 20-second increments until warmed through.

YAFFI'S CLASSIC SLOW COOKER MEATBALLS

`DAIRY-FREE` `GLUTEN-FREE` `NUT-FREE`

YIELD: 20 to 30 meatballs **PREP TIME:** 20 minutes **COOK TIME:** 4 to 6 hours, unattended

1 medium zucchini, chopped

1 medium onion, chopped

1 pound ground beef

1 pound ground turkey

3 large eggs

½ cup gluten-free old-fashioned rolled oats

4 garlic cloves, minced

1 tablespoon dried basil

1 tablespoon dried oregano

1 (25-ounce) jar low-sodium marinara sauce

1 (12-ounce) package whole wheat spaghetti, cooked (optional)

If there is one food my kids demand, it's meatballs and spaghetti. And when it comes to whole wheat pasta, the thinner shapes cook best—for example, spaghetti has better texture than linguini or penne.

1. In a food processor or blender, puree the zucchini with the onion.

2. In a large bowl, combine the beef and turkey, then add the zucchini mixture. Stir in the eggs, oats, garlic, basil, and oregano, and mix until well blended. I like to use a potato masher and set my mixing bowl on a low counter for the best leverage.

3. Using a spoon, form meatballs of about 2 tablespoons each, shaping and rolling the balls as you make them.

4. Pour a thin layer of marinara into the slow cooker. Add half the meatballs to the cooker, then pour in another layer of marinara. Repeat with the remaining meatballs and top with the remaining marinara.

5. Slow-cook on low for 6 hours or on high for 4 hours, until the internal temperature of the meatballs is 165°F.

6. Serve the meatballs over spaghetti, if desired, or on their own.

SUBSTITUTION TIP: If you're not into zucchini, try replacing it with 8 ounces mushrooms (any variety).

STORAGE TIP: Freeze these cooked meatballs for up to 6 months in an airtight container for an easy make-ahead option.

GINGER-GARLIC ROASTED TOFU

DAIRY-FREE **GLUTEN-FREE** **NUT-FREE** **ONE PAN** **VEGAN**

YIELD: 3 (4-ounce/½-cup) servings **PREP TIME:** 5 minutes, plus 20 minutes to marinate
COOK TIME: 20 minutes

3 tablespoons
  pureed Medjool
  dates
1 tablespoon
  toasted sesame oil
2 tablespoons
  coconut amino
  acids or low-
  sodium soy sauce
2 garlic cloves, diced
¼ teaspoon
  ground ginger,
  or ½ teaspoon
  grated
  fresh ginger
1 (14-ounce) block
  firm tofu, pressed
  and cubed
1 tablespoon
  olive oil

Tofu is versatile, inexpensive, and widely available (and keeps well as it waits for its turn in your smoothies or oven). Many people believe that tofu is bland, but it can easily absorb any flavors you add. Start by pressing your tofu in a tofu press or wrap it in paper towels and press under that chemistry book you haven't yet donated. To puree the dates, put them in a bowl and cover with hot water. Let sit for 10 minutes to soften, then drain and blend with some of the soaking water.

1. In a large bowl, mix the date puree, sesame oil, coconut aminos, garlic, and ginger. Marinate the tofu in half the sauce for 20 minutes. Reserve the rest of the sauce for dipping.

2. Preheat the oven to 425°F. Line a baking sheet with aluminum foil and lightly brush it with the olive oil.

3. Lay the tofu on the baking sheet and bake for 10 minutes on each side, until the tofu begins to darken and is firm. Let cool, then serve with the dipping sauce.

NUTRITION TIP: Tofu is a great source of protein and calcium, which are important for growing kids. Consider serving this over rice or alongside some pineapple slaw in a lettuce wrap.

MIXED ROOT-VEGGIE FRIES

GLUTEN-FREE **NUT-FREE** **ONE PAN** **VEGETARIAN**

YIELD: 8 (2-ounce/¼-cup) servings **PREP TIME:** 20 minutes **COOK TIME:** 35 minutes

Olive oil spray
2 pounds mixed carrots, parsnips, and sweet potatoes
1 tablespoon cornstarch (optional)
2 tablespoons olive oil or melted unsalted butter
2 tablespoons grated Parmesan cheese
1 teaspoon dried garlic

Fries seem to pair well with everything, from grilled cheese to a chocolate milkshake. In this version, fries take on a whole new color, with boosted nutritional value to match. To make a rainbow plate of fries, get those beautiful multicolored carrots.

1. Preheat the oven to 425°F. Lightly coat a baking sheet with olive oil spray.

2. Wash the sweet potatoes, scrubbing very well if you are keeping the skin.

3. Cut the vegetables into julienne strips about ¼ inch wide and ¼ inch thick.

4. Place the fries in a large bowl or plastic bag. If using cornstarch, toss the fries with the cornstarch.

5. Arrange the fries on the baking sheet in a single layer. Drizzle with the olive oil or butter, then sprinkle with the cheese and garlic.

6. Bake the fries for 20 minutes, then flip and bake for another 15 minutes, until golden.

NUTRITION TIP: Root vegetables are wonderful sources of fiber. Fiber doesn't only support a healthy bowel pattern; it also feeds the beneficial bacteria that line our large intestines, supporting immunity, cheerful moods, and so much more.

PUMPKIN WHITE BEAN MUFFINS

DAIRY-FREE **GLUTEN-FREE** **VEGAN**

YIELD: 12 muffins PREP TIME: 5 minutes, plus 30 minutes to cool COOK TIME: 20 minutes

Nonstick cooking spray (optional)

½ cup canned pure pumpkin puree or Roasted Butternut Squash Puree (page 29)

2 teaspoons no-alcohol vanilla extract

¼ cup nut or seed butter of choice

1 (15-ounce) can low-sodium white beans, rinsed well and drained

6 Medjool dates, soaked in hot water and drained

½ cup gluten-free old-fashioned rolled oats

¼ teaspoon kosher salt

2 teaspoons ground cinnamon

½ teaspoon baking powder

⅛ teaspoon baking soda

I know, I know. You saw that title and thought "Mmm," followed quickly by a "What?" But I promise, these muffins aren't beany at all. They are fudgy and satisfying. They are also super easy, and muffins are perfect for a little one learning to self-feed, since they are easy to grab. The recipe can be doubled and the baked muffins frozen for up to 3 months—if you have any left to freeze.

1. Preheat the oven to 350°F. Line the cups of a standard 12-cup muffin tin with liners or coat them with cooking spray.

2. Place the pumpkin puree, vanilla, and nut or seed butter in a blender or food processor and blend until smooth.

3. Add the beans, dates, oats, salt, cinnamon, baking powder, and baking soda, and blend until smooth.

4. Fill the muffin cups evenly with the batter, filling each about halfway. Bake for 20 minutes. They will look undercooked, almost like light orange Play-Doh, so don't overbake them.

5. Set the muffins aside to cool and firm up for 30 minutes before enjoying.

NUTRITION TIP: While it's important that your baby not get a lot of salt, including such a small amount in a recipe that yields 12 servings will be fine for your baby's system.

BAKED SALMON CROQUETTES

DAIRY-FREE **NUT-FREE** ONE PAN

YIELD: 8 croquettes **PREP TIME:** 10 minutes **COOK TIME:** 10 to 15 minutes

Nonstick cooking
   spray (optional)
1 (15-ounce) can
   skinless, boneless
   salmon, drained
   and flaked
1½ cups soft
   whole wheat
   bread crumbs
½ cup finely
   chopped red
   bell pepper
3 large eggs,
   lightly beaten
3 green onions,
   white and light
   green parts,
   thinly sliced
¼ cup finely
   chopped celery
¼ cup minced
   fresh cilantro
3 tablespoons
   mayonnaise
1 tablespoon
   lemon juice
1 garlic clove,
   minced

Fatty fish, such as salmon, herring, albacore tuna, and sardines, provide a big boost of omega-3 fatty acids, specifically DHA. DHA is essential for brain growth and development through pregnancy, childhood, and adulthood, as well. This recipe uses canned salmon. Ideally, choose wild-caught salmon that is skinless and boneless. These croquettes are a delicious meal that keeps nicely and travels well, too. If desired, vary the veggies to meet your family's preferences and needs.

1. Preheat the oven to 425°F. Line the cups of an 8-cup muffin tin with muffin liners or coat with cooking spray.

2. In a large bowl, combine the salmon, bread crumbs, bell pepper, eggs, green onions, celery, cilantro, mayonnaise, lemon juice, and garlic; mix until well blended.

3. Pour ⅓ cup of the mixture into each muffin cup.

4. Bake for 10 to 15 minutes, until the internal temperature of the croquette is 160°F.

5. Let cool for 15 to 20 minutes before enjoying.

SUBSTITUTION TIP: You can also use tuna here, but owing to the higher mercury content of albacore tuna, intake should be limited. A standard serving of tuna is 2 ounces (¼ cup). A safer option, according to the EPA and FDA, is to use light tuna, either chunk or solid; it's safe for children to consume one serving per week of light tuna, as opposed to one serving per month of albacore tuna.

BUTTERNUT SQUASH MAC AND CHEESE

NUT-FREE **VEGETARIAN**

YIELD: 8 to 10 servings **PREP TIME:** 20 minutes **COOK TIME:** 50 minutes

1 (16-ounce)
  package pasta
  shells or macaroni
1 tablespoon
  olive oil
Nonstick
  cooking spray
2 tablespoons
  unsalted butter
3 large garlic
  cloves, minced
4 cups diced
  butternut squash,
  or 2 cups Roasted
  Butternut Squash
  Puree (page 29)
1½ cups low- or
  no-sodium
  vegetable broth
2 cups half-and-
  half, divided
8 ounces sharp
  cheddar cheese,
  shredded
¼ cup panko
  bread crumbs
2 tablespoons
  grated Parmesan
  cheese

In this comforting mac and cheese, I increase the amount of vitamin A, vitamin C, and fiber with the addition of the squash. As for the cheese, make sure it is shredded so it melts well; using chunked cheese will result in a lumpy sauce.

1. In a large pot, cook the pasta according to the package instructions until al dente, about 10 minutes. Rinse and drain, but reserve 1 cup of the cooking liquid. Place the pasta in a bowl and stir in the olive oil to prevent the pasta from sticking together.

2. Preheat the oven to 375°F. Coat a 2-quart baking dish with cooking spray.

3. Heat the butter in a large saucepan over medium heat until just starting to brown. Add the garlic and cook for about 1 minute, stirring constantly, until fragrant.

4. Add the diced squash and broth to the saucepan, bring to a simmer, cover, and cook for 10 minutes, until the squash softens.

5. Use an immersion blender to puree the squash until smooth. Alternatively, let the squash cool briefly, then transfer it to a blender or food processor and blend until smooth, adding about ½ cup of the half-and-half to reach the desired consistency.

CONTINUED >

BUTTERNUT SQUASH MAC AND CHEESE CONTINUED

6. Pour the puree back into the saucepan (or add the 2 cups squash puree, if using). Stir in the remaining half-and-half and gently heat the sauce, stirring well. Gradually stir in the cheese, ½ cup at a time, until fully incorporated and creamy.

7. Pour the sauce over the pasta, tossing to combine and using as much of the reserved cooking water to thin as needed. Transfer the pasta and sauce to the baking dish.

8. In a small bowl, mix the bread crumbs and Parmesan cheese, sprinkle it on top of the pasta, and bake for 25 minutes, until bubbly. (If desired, broil for an additional 2 to 3 minutes, until the top is just browned.)

NUTRITION TIP: Add a handful of small fresh broccoli florets before baking to make this mac and cheese colorful and nutritious.

POPCORN ROASTED CAULIFLOWER

DAIRY-FREE GLUTEN-FREE NUT-FREE ONE PAN VEGAN

YIELD: 8 (¼-cup) servings **PREP TIME:** 10 minutes **COOK TIME:** 40 minutes

Nonstick cooking
  spray (optional)
1 head of
  cauliflower
¼ cup olive oil
1 teaspoon
  kosher salt
½ teaspoon
  garlic powder
½ teaspoon
  onion powder

This roasted cauliflower is perfect for the baby who is progressing to simple finger foods or for baby-led weaning! Cauliflower is high in vitamin C, which helps support immunity, and vitamin B_6, excellent for brain development.

1. Preheat the oven to 400°F. Line a baking sheet with parchment paper, or use aluminum foil and lightly it coat with cooking spray.

2. Cut the cauliflower into very small florets, about the size of popped popcorn.

3. In a large bowl, toss the cauliflower with the olive oil, salt, and garlic and onion powders.

4. Spread the cauliflower in a single layer on the baking sheet and bake for 20 minutes, then flip and bake for another 20 minutes, until golden on the outside and soft inside.

5. Let cool briefly and then serve.

MEAL TIP: As an alternative, after baking the cauliflower, drizzle it with the sauce from Butternut Squash Mac and Cheese (page 91) to boost the nutrition and overall food experience.

DEVILISHLY DELICIOUS VEGGIE-STUFFED EGGS

30 MINUTES OR LESS · DAIRY-FREE · GLUTEN-FREE · NUT-FREE · VEGETARIAN

YIELD: 8 servings **PREP TIME:** 10 minutes

4 hard-boiled
   large eggs

3 tablespoons
   mayonnaise

1 tablespoon
   minced red
   bell pepper

1 tablespoon
   minced green
   onion, white and
   light green parts

1 tablespoon
   minced celery

Dash of sweet
   paprika

Hard-boiled eggs are a staple at this age. They are easy to prepare, nutritious, and fun to eat; popping the yolk out of the white never ceases to entertain. Kick it up a notch with these deviled eggs and check out the tips that follow for ways to increase nutrition and color!

1. Peel and then slice the hard-boiled eggs in half lengthwise. Pop out the yolks and place them in a small bowl.

2. Using a fork, smash the yolks, then add the mayo and mix until smooth and creamy.

3. Add the red pepper, green onion, and celery. Mix to incorporate.

4. Using a small spoon, carefully add the yolk mixture back into the white halves.

5. Sprinkle some paprika over the top and enjoy!

NUTRITION TIP: To change up the flavor and nutrition, swap out the mayo with the same amount of flavored hummus. Or consider replacing half the mayo with pesto.

FRENCH TOAST STRIPS

30 MINUTES OR LESS **NUT-FREE** **ONE PAN** **VEGETARIAN**

YIELD: 16 strips **PREP TIME:** 10 minutes **COOK TIME:** 4 to 6 minutes

2 large eggs

1 teaspoon
no-alcohol
vanilla extract

½ teaspoon ground
cinnamon

2 tablespoons cow's
milk or non-dairy
alternative

4 slices bread
of choice

1 tablespoon
unsalted butter
(optional)

Fresh berries or
Roasted Banana
Puree (page 25),
for serving

When you think of the ingredients for French toast—bread, eggs, and milk—it's easy to see it as a nutrition-friendly option. I use an electric griddle set at 300°F, which makes it nearly impossible to burn your breakfast while chasing a toddler or changing a diaper, but it's also easily made in a skillet.

1. In a medium bowl, beat the eggs with the vanilla, cinnamon, and milk.

2. Cut each bread slice into 4 strips, then soak each strip in the egg mixture for 2 to 3 minutes, poking a hole in each piece as it soaks. Place the strips back in the bowl, spreading them out as much as possible. When you're ready to cook, place a plate over the bowl and carefully flip everything upside down; this way, the strips that have been soaking the longest are the first cooked, while the final strips will continue to absorb more liquid.

3. If using an electric griddle, set it to 300°F. If using a skillet, heat a teaspoon of the butter over medium heat. When the griddle or skillet is hot, cook the strips for 2 to 3 minutes on each side, until golden brown. If using the skillet, you may need to add more butter between batches.

4. Serve the strips along with some fresh berries or with Roasted Banana Puree.

MAKE-AHEAD TIP: After cooking, allow the strips to cool completely, then place them in a freezer-safe, airtight container for up to a month. When ready to enjoy, and toast the frozen strips on a griddle or in a skillet.

MICROWAVED PORRIDGE FINGERS

30 MINUTES OR LESS | **GLUTEN-FREE** | **NUT-FREE** | **ONE PAN** | **VEGETARIAN**

YIELD: 8 to 12 fingers **PREP TIME:** 5 minutes, plus 20 minutes to soak **COOK TIME:** 2 minutes

4 tablespoons gluten-free old-fashioned rolled oats

2 tablespoons cow's milk or non-dairy alternative

2 tablespoons applesauce

1 tablespoon peeled and grated fresh apple

½ teaspoon ground cinnamon

Porridge is a classic breakfast. You can dress it up or dress it down. But no matter how you enjoy it, it will keep baby full and satisfied long into the day. These porridge fingers travel well and are easily accepted by tiny taste buds. This recipe is a bit mild and will appeal more to littles than to adults, as babies pick up on the very subtle flavors we often miss as adults.

1. Mix the oats, milk, and applesauce in a medium bowl. Soak until mushy, about 20 minutes.

2. Stir in the grated apple and cinnamon.

3. Press the mixture into a 9-by-13-inch baking dish using the back of a spoon.

4. Microwave on high for 2 minutes.

5. Cut into strips while still hot, then let cool to room temperature before serving.

ADDITION TIP: Consider adding some flavor to represent the season; for example, add blueberries in the summer, pumpkin pie spice in the fall (replacing the cinnamon), shaved dark chocolate in the winter, and cherries in the spring.

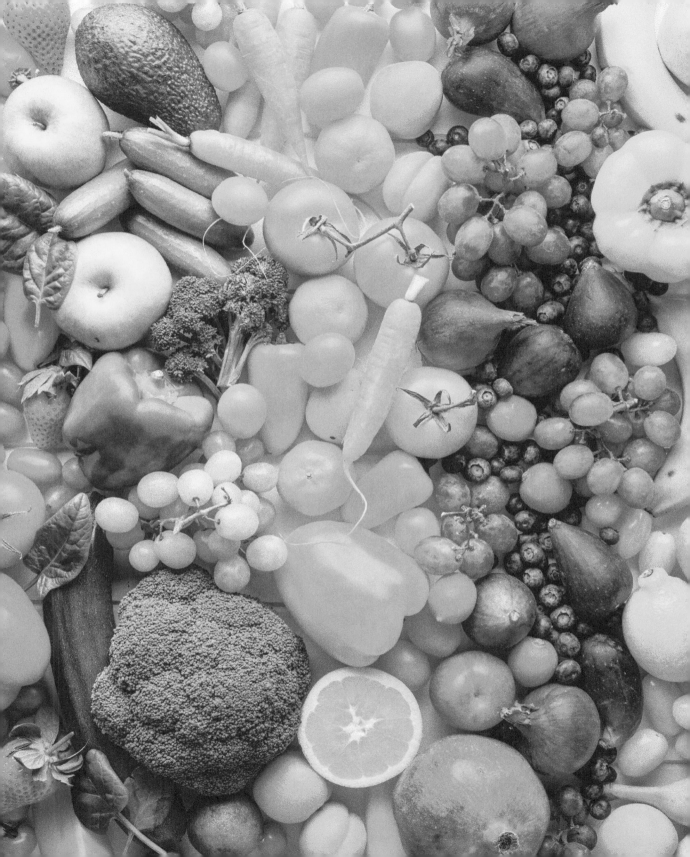

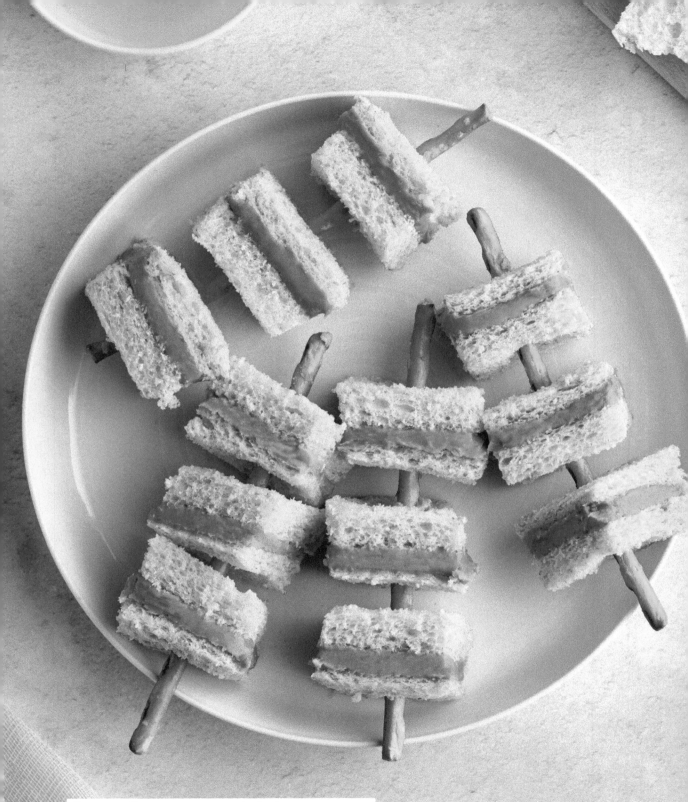

PEANUT BUTTER SANDWICH KEBABS PAGE 105

5

12 TO 18 MONTHS

TODDLER MEALS

OPTIMAL NUTRITION

Your baby is now at the point of depending on food for nutrition rather than on breast milk or formula. Watch for your child's reaction to new foods. A baby may make a "yuck" face but still go back for more. Allow your child to explore new flavor sensations as you explore these with them! This is also the time to invite your little one into the kitchen to start helping to create delicious masterpieces alongside their favorite chef—you!

When in doubt, add something nutritious to baby's plate.

NEW LIQUIDS FOR BABY

At this age, there are many beverage options. There is a lot of confusion regarding this transition, so here's the straight talk (no milk chaser).

Transitioning to Milk

If you've been breastfeeding, you now have the option of weaning. If you do choose to continue breastfeeding, your breast milk remains a nutritious option, either in place of or alongside cow's milk or a non-dairy alternative milk.

If you've been using formula, you are free to quit! You can transition directly to milk at this point. However, if you notice that your child is experiencing tummy discomfort, you can make that transition more slowly. Mix expressed breast milk or formula with cow's milk; for example, 25 percent cow's milk and 75 percent breast milk or formula, then go to 50/50, then to 75/25, and finally to 100 percent cow's milk. This transition can take one to two weeks, depending on your child. If you are transitioning to a non-dairy milk, you can use the same transition method.

If you are transitioning to cow's milk, select whole milk. The fat in whole milk is full of nutrition and is especially beneficial for brain growth. If you're transitioning to non-dairy milk, select an alternative plant-based milk that is fortified with calcium. Many non-dairy milks are short on, or even devoid of, fat, so you'll need to make that up in another area of your child's food intake. Soy milk is a great alternative because it naturally contains some fat and protein. Whole soy products, including soy milk, tofu, soy sauce, and edamame, are perfectly safe for your little one.

While cow's milk is fortified with vitamin D, the fortification doesn't meet the levels that the American Academy of Pediatrics recommends, so continue to supplement your child with 400 IU of vitamin D daily.

Incorporating Water and Juice

At this point, water is important for hydration and should be offered at and between all meals. If your child doesn't find water interesting, consider adding whole chunks of fruit, like pineapple, strawberries, melon, cucumber, or even mint, to improve the taste.

If a child is constipated, it may be beneficial to use 2 to 4 ounces (¼ to ½ cup) of pure pear or prune juice to help produce a bowel movement, but this should be considered medicinal. For now, it's best to avoid juice as a beverage, owing to the high sugar content and lack of fiber. As your child grows and becomes social, they may be in a situation where juice is offered. It's okay to allow your child to socialize by participating with the other children. Putting a "forbidden" label on juices (and other foods) will likely make it more alluring to your child.

IMPORTANT NUTRIENTS

Solid food now comes before the breast or bottle, both in timing and in nutritional importance. While nutrition is important at this stage, your baby will not be expected to meet their nutrition needs at a single meal, or even in a single day. Children, as well as adults, meet their nutrition needs over the course of a few days. There is no need to count bites or pressure your child to eat more of a certain food or less of another food. You will present the food and set the mood!

FOODS TO EMBRACE

Your baby's kidneys and immune system are now mature enough to handle salt and honey. You may choose to continue cooking with minimal salt, but the occasional slice of store-bought pizza or take-out food is fine (and is sometimes necessary for sanity).

Each meal should include a protein, a vegetable and/or fruit, and a starch. There should always be a "safe" option—an item of food that is often accepted and enjoyed by the child (see page 104)—on the table.

At this point, there is no single food that should be avoided unless your child has a food allergy. Your pediatrician can advise on how and when to reintroduce a food that was previously an allergen, but it's important to know that many childhood allergies will be outgrown, particularly allergies to cow's milk, wheat, and eggs.

While added sugar isn't dangerous, try to wait until age 2 to introduce your little one to very sugary foods. When you have a single child, it's easy to avoid added sugars, but when older siblings are enjoying a sweet treat in front of your littlest one, allow them to participate. Restriction could result in a child who actively prefers—and seeks out—sweets. By calmly allowing the child to participate, you will send the message that dessert isn't anything special. This neutralizes the overall method, effectively avoiding the delicious and enticing "forbidden" label that comes with a side of long-term sugar obsession.

TYPICAL TOOLS AND UTENSILS

While your little one will still benefit from the same utensils you've been using (see page 11), it might be time to expand your tool chest! Cooking with your kids is a great way to gently expose them to new foods in a pressure-free way. Buy a child-safe knife, such as the ones offered by Curious Chef or Tovla. While bringing food prep down to the floor is always an option, having a Learning Tower can be a useful tool to bring your little chef to the countertop safely and securely.

TYPICAL MEALS AND SCHEDULE

Every family has a different dynamic, and therefore a different schedule. Starting at 12 months, your schedule might resemble the one on the facing page. Awake time between naps will be two, three, and four hours as the day progresses.

Sample Meal Schedule

6:00 A.M.	Wake up
6:30 A.M.	Breakfast; include 2 ounces (¼ cup) whole milk
8:00 A.M.	Morning nap (45 to 60 minutes or more is great)
9:15 A.M.	Snack 1; include 2 ounces (¼ cup) whole milk
11:30 A.M.	Lunch; include 2 ounces (¼ cup) whole milk
12:00 P.M.	Nap (1½ to 2 hours or more)
2:30 P.M.	Snack 2; include 2 ounces (¼ cup) whole milk
5:00 P.M.	Dinner; include 2 ounces (¼ cup) whole milk
6:00 P.M.	Bedtime

COMMON CHALLENGES

Here are some common challenges at this stage.

MY CHILD IS PICKY.

The primary obstacle that parents of children at this age report is "pickiness." I choose to say that these kids are "selective," "cautious," or "hesitant," because this is just a phase. The words I choose are softer and have a temporary connotation, whereas "picky" can sound harsh and more permanent. If a child hears you calling them "picky," they will own it.

When kids become more independently mobile, as they take their first steps, the risk increases drastically that they will inadvertently eat something dangerous. There is a corresponding biological response that tells them to be less curious and more cautious. There are proactive steps you can take to ensure ongoing curiosity with food:

1. **COOK WITH YOUR CHILD.** For a full cooking experience, check out my book *Fun with Food Toddler Cookbook*. Bring your little chef into the kitchen to make an Orange Dreamsicle Smoothie (page 77) or Avocado Muffins (page 117). Give them a potato masher, kid-safe chef's knife, or peeler and watch what they can accomplish.

2. **START AN HERB GARDEN.** Place the little pots of herbs on your windowsill and watch your child's wonder as the aromatic and delicious herbs take root and grow—just like your child is growing.

3. **FOLLOW THE DIVISION OF RESPONSIBILITY.** This is a responsive feeding dynamic whereby the parent is in charge of what is served, where it is served, and when it is served. The child is in charge of whether or not they will eat and how much. While you as parent decide what to serve for a meal or a snack, always include a "safe" food item that you know your child loves. See more learning options in the Resources (page 154).

PEANUT BUTTER SANDWICH KEBABS

30 MINUTES OR LESS | **DAIRY-FREE** | **VEGAN**

YIELD: 4 kebabs **PREP TIME:** 10 minutes

2 slices whole wheat bread

1 tablespoon natural peanut butter or other nut butter

4 unsalted pretzel sticks

Anyone who has been to a state fair knows that everything tastes better on a stick. This recipe takes the classic peanut butter sandwich and skewers it, making a fun and delicious meal or snack. The ice-pop sticks or wooden coffee stirrers I would normally advise will not work for this age, so unsalted pretzel sticks make a great stand-in until your little one gets a bit bigger.

1. Use the bread and peanut butter to make a sandwich.

2. Cut the sandwich into 12 squares.

3. Skewer 4 squares carefully onto each of the pretzel sticks! Depending on the density of your bread, it may be helpful to first skewer your squares with a chopstick to create room for the pretzel.

COOKING TIP: Did you know that you don't actually have to stir natural peanut butter before you use it? You can just store it upside down in the refrigerator for a day prior to opening it. The oil will recombine with the peanut butter and you can enjoy all the health benefits of that oil without a mess.

ALMOND MEAL PANCAKES

NUT-FREE **ONE PAN** **VEGETARIAN**

YIELD: 15 pancakes **PREP TIME:** 10 minutes **COOK TIME:** 30 to 40 minutes

1 cup whole
   wheat flour
½ cup almond meal
   or almond flour
1 tablespoon
   baking powder
½ teaspoon
   kosher salt
4 Medjool dates,
   pitted and pureed
1¼ cups cow's
   milk or non-dairy
   alternative
1 large egg,
   lightly beaten
3 tablespoons
   unsalted butter,
   melted
Nonstick cooking
   spray (optional)

These pancakes are the perfect comfort food on a lazy Sunday morning. If desired, double the recipe and freeze the extras. I use an electric griddle, but you can also make these in a skillet.

1. Mix the flour, almond meal, baking powder, and salt in a large bowl. Form a well in the center of the dry mixture.

2. In a small bowl, combine the dates, milk, egg, and melted butter.

3. Pour the wet ingredients into the well and stir just until incorporated and smooth. Allow the batter to sit for 5 minutes.

4. Meanwhile, heat an electric griddle to 300°F or coat a large skillet with cooking spray. When the griddle or skillet is hot, pour ¼ cup of batter onto the surface and cook until tiny bubbles appear on the surface, about 3 minutes. Flip the pancake and cook another 2 minutes, until golden. Keep the pancake warm while you make the remaining pancakes, then serve.

MEAL TIP: Serve these pancakes with plain full-fat Greek yogurt and Roasted Pear and Date Puree (page 66) for a super-fancy experience.

EASY VEGGIE AND TOFU SCRAMBLE

30 MINUTES OR LESS **DAIRY-FREE** **GLUTEN-FREE** **NUT-FREE** **ONE PAN** **VEGAN**

YIELD: 4 to 6 servings **PREP TIME:** 5 minutes **COOK TIME:** 20 minutes

Pinch of kosher salt

¼ teaspoon ground turmeric

¼ teaspoon ground cumin (optional)

2 tablespoons olive oil

1 garlic clove, minced

¼ medium onion, thinly sliced

½ bell pepper, thinly sliced

2 cups (packed) chopped fresh spinach, kale, dandelion greens, or a mixture

8 ounce extra-firm tofu

What is easier than scrambled eggs? Not much. But what if you're vegan? Have an egg allergy? Try the tofu twist and you may never look back! This tofu scramble can be dressed up or served simply with a side of berries or toast.

1. Combine the salt, turmeric, and cumin (if using) in a small bowl. Add just enough water (about a tablespoon) to create a light sauce.

2. Heat the olive oil in a large skillet over medium heat. Add the garlic, onion, and bell pepper and sauté for 4 to 5 minutes, until beginning to soften.

3. Add the greens, cover, turn off the heat, and let sit for 1 to 2 minutes, until the greens begin to wilt.

4. Crumble the tofu into the pan and set it over medium heat. Cook, stirring, for 2 minutes.

5. Add the reserved sauce, stir once, and cook for another 5 to 7 minutes, stirring occasionally. The mixture will look yellow-brown, kind of like traditional scrambled eggs. Allow to cool to a temperature appropriate for your child and serve.

NUTRITION TIP: Don't fear sharp tastes! Your baby has been experiencing the world through taste since the womb. Adding strong flavors like onion and bell pepper can improve their meal experience, creating a positive table environment.

CARROT CAKE WAFFLES

30 MINUTES OR LESS | **NUT-FREE** | **VEGETARIAN**

YIELD: 4 thick waffles **PREP TIME:** 10 minutes **COOK TIME:** 15 minutes

1 cup whole
wheat flour

¾ cups old-
fashioned
rolled oats

1 tablespoon
baking powder

2 teaspoon ground
cinnamon

¼ cup cornstarch

Pinch of
ground nutmeg

¼ teaspoon
kosher salt

2 large eggs,
lightly beaten

3 Medjool dates,
pitted and pureed

1½ teaspoons
no-alcohol
vanilla extract

½ cup olive or
avocado oil

1¾ cups cow's
milk or non-dairy
alternative

3 medium carrots,
shredded

⅓ cup raisins
(optional)

This is a fancy and decadent breakfast, and if made ahead will keep well in the freezer for up to 3 months. These Belgian-style waffles feature the comforting flavors of carrot cake to produce a unique and nutritious breakfast.

1. Preheat a waffle iron.

2. In a large bowl, combine the flour, oats, baking powder, cinnamon, cornstarch, nutmeg, and salt. Create a well in the middle of the dry mixture.

3. Add the eggs, dates, vanilla, oil, and milk to the well. Mix just to incorporate, then fold in the carrots and raisins (if using).

4. Pour one-quarter of the batter onto the waffle iron, close, and cook for approximately 3 minutes, following the manufacturer's instructions. Remove and keep waffle warm while you make the remaining 3 waffles. To serve, cut the waffles into pieces for your child to enjoy.

NUTRITION TIP: Carrots contain beta-carotene, which needs fat to be fully absorbed. Consider pairing this breakfast with a spoonful of some full-fat Greek yogurt and a handful of finely chopped nuts on top to reap all those benefits.

FRUIT AND YOGURT PARFAITS

30 MINUTES OR LESS | VEGETARIAN

YIELD: 2 to 4 servings **PREP TIME:** 5 minutes

1 cup plain full-fat Greek yogurt or non-dairy alternative

1 cup mixed fresh or frozen berries

Toppings of choice: ½ cup granola, crushed nuts, shredded coconut, and/or sliced banana

Parfait is a French word meaning "perfect." And these parfaits are perfect because that's exactly what you were craving! To increase the fun, use transparent dishes so the layers are visible.

Layer the yogurt, berries, and toppings in 2 medium or 4 small cups or bowls.

ADDITION TIP: You can vary this by substituting cottage cheese or even the Overnight Chia Pudding (page 64). Also, consider adding a layer of one of these purees: Mixed Berry (page 23), Roasted Banana (page 25), Melon (page 24), or Peach (page 26).

BROCCOLI AND CHEDDAR QUINOA CUPS

GLUTEN-FREE NUT-FREE ONE PAN VEGETARIAN

YIELD: 8 quinoa cups **PREP TIME:** 10 minutes **COOK TIME:** 20 minutes

Nonstick cooking
   spray (optional)
1 tablespoon
   unsalted butter, at
   room temperature
4 large eggs,
   lightly beaten
3 tablespoons cow's
   milk or non-dairy
   alternative
1 cup cooked
   quinoa
¾ cup shredded
   cheddar cheese
½ cup chopped
   fresh or frozen
   broccoli florets,
   thawed if frozen

I don't know about you, but I sure love broccoli. It's bright green, it looks like little trees, and it's so delicious. These quinoa cups make a wonderful breakfast, lunch, dinner, or snack, and they are great for using up leftover quinoa. This may look like kid food, but be sure to try one yourself. You may not be able to stop at just one.

1. Preheat the oven to 375°F. Coat an 8-cup muffin tin with cooking spray or line the cups with muffin liners.

2. Combine the butter, eggs, milk, quinoa, cheese, and broccoli in a large bowl.

3. Divide the mixture evenly among the muffin cups and bake for 20 minutes, or until golden brown.

4. Let the quinoa cups stand for 5 to 10 minutes before releasing them from the tin and serving.

ADDITION TIP: Add 1 minced garlic clove to the mix to kick up the flavor!

NUTRITION TIP: Quinoa is a good source of protein and fiber, but the best benefit at this stage is in exposing your child to unfamiliar textures.

HOME-COOKED FISH STICKS

`30 MINUTES OR LESS` `DAIRY-FREE` `NUT-FREE` `ONE PAN`

YIELD: 10 to 12 fish sticks **PREP TIME:** 10 minutes **COOK TIME:** 15 minutes

Nonstick cooking
   spray (optional)
1 cup panko
   bread crumbs
½ teaspoon
   kosher salt
1 teaspoon sweet or
   smoked paprika
1 teaspoon lemon
   pepper seasoning
Grated zest and
   juice of 1 lemon
   (1 tablespoon zest
   and 2 tablespoons
   lemon juice)
2 large eggs,
   lightly beaten
1 cup all-purpose
   flour
1½ pounds white
   fish fillets (such
   as tilapia, catfish,
   trout, pollock, or
   cod), cut into
   1-inch strips

Fish sticks are a childhood classic. Since these are freezer-friendly for up to 3 months, you can make a few batches and freeze them, unbaked, for that one day when you're stuck in traffic or that time when you'd just prefer to take a sunset bike ride rather than prepare dinner. I've been there. Choose the bike ride.

1. Preheat the oven to 400°F. Liberally coat a baking sheet with cooking spray or line it with parchment paper.

2. In a small bowl, combine the bread crumbs, salt, paprika, lemon pepper, and lemon zest.

3. In another small bowl, beat the eggs and lemon juice together.

4. Place the flour into another small bowl.

5. Dip each strip of fish in the flour, shake off any excess, then dip them in the beaten egg, and then in the crumb mixture. Pat the fish as you go to ensure the coating stays on each piece.

6. Place the fish sticks on the baking sheet and bake for 6 minutes. Flip and bake for another 5 to 7 minutes, until both sides are golden brown and flaky.

NUTRITION TIP: Your choice of fish may depend on what is in season, what is on sale, or possibly the level of mercury in each type of fish. The fish suggested within the recipe are all on the low-mercury list provided by the FDA and EPA. See the Resources (page 154) for more information.

RED LENTIL KOFTA CAKES

NUT-FREE **VEGETARIAN**

YIELD: 12 cakes **PREP TIME:** 15 minutes **COOK TIME:** 35 minutes

2 tablespoons
unsalted butter or
olive oil

1 medium
white onion,
chopped small

1 medium carrot,
chopped small

1 tablespoon
tomato paste

2 teaspoons sweet
or smoked paprika

1 teaspoon
ground cumin

1 cup red lentils

2 cups water

1 cup fine bulghur

Nonstick cooking
spray

¾ cup all-purpose
flour

Kofta is a traditional dish in the Middle East and North Africa. In this vegetarian version, the meat is replaced with red lentils. Although the dish comes from my own culture, I didn't know these flavors as a child, but as I grew up and met people of a similar background, I fell in love with this flavor palate. This is my comfort food.

1. Heat a medium saucepan over medium heat. Add the butter and heat until just beginning to brown. Add the onion and carrot, and sauté until soft, about 5 minutes.

2. Stir in the tomato paste, paprika, cumin, red lentils, and water. Simmer over medium heat for 7 to 9 minutes, or until the lentils are soft.

3. Stir in the bulghur and remove from the heat. Let stand for about 20 minutes, until the bulghur is softened.

4. Spread the mixture evenly in a large platter or on a baking sheet to cool.

5. Preheat the oven to 350°F.

6. Coat a standard 12-cup muffin tin with cooking spray. Using a tablespoon measure, scoop up a heaping tablespoon of the mixture and gently form it into a ball. Place it in a muffin cup and gently press to flatten it and cover the bottom of the cup. Lightly coat the top with cooking spray. Repeat with the remaining mixture to fill all the muffin cups.

7. Bake for 15 to 17 minutes, then let cool for 5 minutes before releasing the cakes from the tin.

ADDITION TIP: These little cakes are generally served with a traditional Middle Eastern cucumber and tomato salad, dressed with a squeeze of lemon. You can kick this salad up a notch by adding finely chopped red onion and some minced parsley; just be sure to remove any choking hazard by finely chopping the cucumber and tomato.

SWEET POTATO TOASTS

GLUTEN-FREE NUT-FREE ONE PAN VEGETARIAN

YIELD: 3 toasts **PREP TIME:** 10 minutes **COOK TIME:** 20 minutes

Nonstick cooking
  spray (optional)
1 large sweet potato
3 tablespoons
  full-fat ricotta
3 tablespoons fresh
  or frozen berries

This popular snack made the rounds a few years ago. I just love food fads because they are a way of trying something you haven't yet had or directing you to reimagine a favorite in a new light. Serving sweet potato slices as toast boosts the flavor of your breakfast, increasing the satisfaction quotient.

1. Preheat the oven to 400°F. Line a baking sheet with parchment paper, or use aluminum foil and coat it with cooking spray.

2. Trim the sweet potato, cutting off both ends, and then cut it into ½-inch-thick slices.

3. Place the sweet potato slices on the baking sheet, separating them by at least 1 inch. Bake for 20 minutes, until soft enough to bite, but firm enough to hold any delicious toppings.

4. Let cool for 3 to 5 minutes, then spread with the ricotta and top with the berries.

ADDITION TIP: While a sweet potato slice is delicious, this presentation is only one option. Consider topping the slices with avocado or guacamole, hummus, scrambled or fried egg, cream cheese, or even peanut butter and banana slices.

SPINACH AND ZUCCHINI BAKED FRITTATA

GLUTEN-FREE **NUT-FREE** **ONE PAN** **VEGETARIAN**

YIELD: 8 to 10 slices **PREP TIME:** 10 minutes **COOK TIME:** 30 minutes

3 tablespoons
  unsalted butter

1 cup spiralized or
  chopped fresh
  zucchini

1 medium onion,
  thinly sliced

1 cup (packed)
  chopped
  fresh spinach

12 large eggs,
  lightly beaten

3 tablespoons cow's
  milk or non-dairy
  alternative

3 tablespoons
  sour cream
  or non-dairy
  alternative

½ cup shredded
  or crumbled
  cheddar cheese

½ teaspoon kosher
  salt

This sounds like the perfect fancy dinner, but it's not. It's simply a perfect dinner. It's for the evening after a tough day, the meal for when you're in a hurry, or just the dinner for when you are taking a well-deserved break. If desired, serve it with garlic bread. Using spiralized zucchini gives it a beautiful texture, but you can certainly chop the zucchini instead.

1. In a large ovenproof skillet, such as cast iron, melt the butter over medium heat, then add the zucchini and onion and cook for 5 minutes, until the onion begins to look translucent. Add the spinach and stir until just combined, then remove from heat. Let the spinach wilt.

2. Preheat the oven to 375°F.

3. In a large bowl, whisk together the eggs, milk, sour cream, cheese, and salt. Pour over the vegetables in the skillet.

4. Bake for 20 to 25 minutes, until the eggs look puffed and the center jiggles just a bit. Let cool slightly before slicing and serving.

MAKE-AHEAD TIP: You can prep this ahead up to baking, then cover and refrigerate it for up to 2 days. When ready, just uncover and pop the frittata in a preheated oven and you'll have dinner shortly!

ELOTE (MEXICAN STREET CORN)

30 MINUTES OR LESS **GLUTEN-FREE** **NUT-FREE** **ONE PAN** **VEGETARIAN**

YIELD: 8 to 10 servings **PREP TIME:** 10 minutes **COOK TIME:** 5 minutes

5 ears of corn, shucked, or 3¾ cups frozen corn kernels
½ cup unsalted butter, in pieces, at room temperature
1 cup fresh lime juice
1¼ cups crema Mexicana, crème fraîche, or sour cream
½ cup crumbled cotija cheese or feta

Elote en vaso, or "corn in a cup," is a traditional treat sold in Mexico and in US border cities. As street food, it is often served in a Styrofoam cup. The word *elote* is from the Nahuatl word *elotitutl* and refers to indigenous peoples' staple crop.

1. Place the corn kernels in a large saucepan, cover with water, and bring to a boil. Reduce to a simmer and cook for 2 to 3 minutes, until the corn is soft.

2. Drain the corn and immediately transfer it to a large bowl. Add the butter and stir until melted. Stir in the lime juice and crema.

3. Divide the mixture among small serving dishes and top with the cotija.

NUTRITION TIP: Corn is high in fiber as well as thiamine and folate. It can help maintain a healthy digestive tract while supporting brain growth and development; it also helps the body process food into energy.

AVOCADO MUFFINS

NUT-FREE **VEGETARIAN**

YIELD: 12 muffins **PREP TIME:** 15 minutes **COOK TIME:** 30 minutes

Nonstick cooking
  spray (optional)
2 tablespoons
  chia seeds
4 tablespoons
  hot water
⅓ cup old-fashioned
  rolled oats
1 cup whole
  wheat flour
1 teaspoon
  baking powder
½ teaspoon
  baking soda
½ teaspoon
  kosher salt
1 teaspoon ground
  cinnamon
1 ripe avocado
2 ripe to overripe
  medium bananas
6 Medjool dates,
  pitted
¼ cup olive oil
¼ cup cow's milk
  or non-dairy
  alternative
1 teaspoon fresh
  lemon juice

In this recipe, avocado is the fat that holds it all together. Avocado is full of anti-inflammatory monounsaturated fats, which can help prevent heart disease, cancer, and many other types of illnesses.

1. Preheat the oven to 350°F. Line a standard 12-cup muffin tin with parchment liners or coat with cooking spray.

2. In a small cup, combine the chia seeds and hot water, stir, and let sit for 10 minutes.

3. In a large bowl, combine the oats, flour, baking powder, baking soda, salt, and cinnamon.

4. In a medium bowl, mash the avocado and bananas.

5. Using a blender or mini food processor, blend the dates with the olive oil, then add to the avocado-banana mixture. Stir in the chia. Add the milk and lemon juice and stir again.

6. Add the wet ingredients to the dry ingredients and stir until just combined.

7. Spoon the batter evenly into the muffin cups, filling each cup about three-quarters full.

8. Bake for 30 minutes, until a toothpick inserted in a muffin comes out clean.

COOKING TIP: To make avocado "bread" instead of muffins, pour the batter into an 8-by-4-inch greased loaf pan and bake for 1 hour, or until a toothpick inserted in the center comes out clean.

SIMPLE HOMESTYLE CHICKEN NUGGETS

30 MINUTES OR LESS | DAIRY-FREE | NUT-FREE | ONE PAN

YIELD: 32 nuggets   PREP TIME: 15 minutes   COOK TIME: 15 minutes

Nonstick cooking
 spray (optional)
1½ cups panko
 or whole wheat
 bread crumbs
¼ teaspoon
 onion powder
½ teaspoon
 kosher salt
1 pound ground
 chicken or turkey
1 large egg, lightly
 beaten

Chicken nuggets are considered a childhood classic, but we all know they are great for adults, too. Many of us have fond memories of the chicken nuggets of our childhood, and we can relive those fun times with each bite. Why not pass on the fun to the next generation? Once cooked, these can be frozen for up to 6 months and reheated for a quick and convenient dinner.

1. Preheat the oven to 375°F. Line a baking sheet with parchment paper or use aluminum foil and coat it with cooking spray.

2. Combine the bread crumbs, onion powder, and salt in a medium mixing bowl.

3. In another medium bowl, mix the ground meat and egg.

4. Using a tablespoon, scoop up the ground meat and shape it into balls, then press each into a nugget-shape, about ½ inch thick.

5. Roll each nugget in the crumb mixture until well coated and arrange them on the baking sheet.

6. Lightly spray the nuggets with cooking spray, then bake for 15 minutes, flipping them over halfway through, until golden.

NUTRITION TIP: Dips can be a wonderful additional source of nutrition, as well as fun, and chicken nuggets taste amazing with hummus. Try a plain hummus or a fun variety like red pepper or roasted garlic to boost the flavor while increasing the protein, fiber, and folate, and adding a whole lot more goodness.

RICOTTA PANCAKES

YIELD: 6 to 8 pancakes **PREP TIME:** 5 minutes **COOK TIME:** 25 minutes

3 large eggs

1 cup ricotta

1 teaspoon
no-alcohol
vanilla extract

½ cup all-purpose
flour

1 teaspoon
baking powder

¼ teaspoon
kosher salt

Nonstick cooking
spray (optional)

1 tablespoon
unsalted butter
(optional)

Ricotta has a natural sweetness and a smooth texture that lends itself well to pancake batter. These pancakes are high in protein, while also providing the calcium and fat so important for growth and development. You can double or even triple the recipe, and freeze them for later, up to 3 months!

1. Mix the eggs, ricotta, and vanilla in a medium mixing bowl.

2. Add the flour, baking powder, and salt, and whisk until just combined. Do not overmix.

3. Preheat an electric griddle to 300°F and lightly coat with cooking spray or heat a large skillet over medium heat and add the butter and heat until melted.

4. Using a ¼-cup measure, scoop out some batter and pour it on the griddle or in the skillet. Cook the pancake for 2 to 3 minutes on each side, until golden. Remove and keep warm while you make the remaining pancakes.

MEAL TIP: Consider boosting the flavor and nutrition by serving these pancakes with a sweet puree such as Melon Puree (page 24) or Dried Apricot Puree (page 27).

ONIGIRI (JAPANESE RICE BALLS)

30 MINUTES OR LESS | **DAIRY-FREE** | **GLUTEN-FREE** | **NUT-FREE**

YIELD: 4 to 6 rice balls **PREP TIME:** 10 minutes

1 cup steamed
   sushi rice
Pinch of kosher salt
4 tablespoons tuna
   salad or other
   filling of choice
2 tablespoons
   black or white
   sesame seeds

Japanese rice balls are called both *onigiri* and *omusubi*, and are a staple of Bento boxes. The one change I've made, for choking hazard reasons, is to skip the nori that usually wraps the rice balls. Instead, I opt for the equally traditional but baby-friendlier sesame seed coating.

1. Wet your hands to prevent sticking and rub them with some salt. Using about 2 tablespoons of rice, shape and press a ball that feels dense.

2. Push 1½ teaspoons of the filling into the ball and close the rice around the filling, shaping a smooth ball.

3. Spread the seeds on a wide dish, then roll the rice ball in the sesame seeds to coat. Set aside.

4. Repeat until all the rice and filling are used.

SUBSTITUTION TIP: This recipe gives you the basics, but it's traditional to stuff rice balls with a savory or sweet treat, such as grilled salmon flakes or pickled plum. I like to fill mine with baked salmon.

TRADITIONAL MAC AND CHEESE

30 MINUTES OR LESS | NUT-FREE | VEGETARIAN

YIELD: 4 to 6 servings **PREP TIME:** 5 minutes **COOK TIME:** 10 minutes

2 cups cow's milk
or non-dairy
alternative

⅓ cup unsalted
butter

⅓ cup all-purpose
flour

¾ teaspoon
kosher salt

Freshly ground
black pepper

2 cups shredded
sharp cheddar
cheese

2 cups cooked
macaroni

What's more comforting than a creamy mac and cheese? It is economical and widely accepted, and provides an easy base for a nutritious meal. You can serve this on the side of a more substantial menu or add vegetables to increase color, vary the texture, and boost the nutrition.

1. Warm the milk in a medium saucepan over low heat until little bubbles appear, about 2 minutes. Turn off the heat.

2. In a large saucepan, melt the butter. Stir in the flour and cook, stirring consistently, until the mixture bubbles a bit. Don't let it brown. This will take about 2 minutes.

3. Add the hot milk, stir, and bring to a boil. Add salt and pepper. Lower the heat and cook for 2 to 3 more minutes, until it thickens.

4. Slowly add the cheese, still stirring, until combined and smooth.

5. Add the macaroni to the saucepan, stir well, and serve.

ADDITION TIP: Just as for the Butternut Squash Mac and Cheese on page 91, you can add roasted broccoli here, too. You might also consider adding rinsed and drained canned black beans and some mild salsa for a Southwest feeling, or canned light tuna and frozen peas, leftover Thanksgiving turkey, or even roasted Brussels sprouts and butternut squash.

VEGGIE STIR-FRY

30 MINUTES OR LESS | DAIRY-FREE | NUT-FREE | ONE PAN | VEGETARIAN

YIELD: 4 to 6 servings   **PREP TIME:** 5 minutes   **COOK TIME:** 10 minutes

2 Medjool dates,
   pitted and pureed
1 tablespoon
   toasted sesame oil
2 tablespoons
   low-sodium soy
   sauce or tamari
2 garlic cloves, diced
¼ teaspoon
   ground ginger, or
   ½ teaspoon grated
   fresh ginger
1 tablespoon
   olive oil
2 cups cooked rice
   or quinoa
1 to 2 cups mixed
   cooked fresh or
   frozen vegetables
1 large egg
   (optional)

You can toss so many leftovers into a stir-fry. A common complaint about feeding kids is the food waste. So, consider food waste as you might the many sheets of paper on which your child will practice handwriting. Just as you wouldn't think of that paper as wasted, as it's part of learning a new skill, the food waste is simply the normal and expected result when a child is learning how to eat. But unlike paper, you can sometimes repurpose the leftovers into something new and delicious.

1. Combine the date puree, sesame oil, soy sauce, garlic, and ginger in a small bowl. Set aside.

2. In a large sauté pan, heat the olive oil, then add the rice. Stir to coat well, then add the vegetables. Cook for 2 to 3 minutes, until everything is hot.

3. Drizzle in the sauce to taste and stir.

4. If desired, crack the egg directly onto the mixture and stir-fry until cooked, 2 to 3 minutes.

5. Let cool slightly and serve.

ADDITION TIP: Consider adding sweet peas, asparagus, green beans, bell peppers, broccoli, mushrooms, onions, or zucchini to your stir-fry. Steam or sauté before starting step 1 so you can be sure that the vegetables will be just a little crunchy when joining the party in the pan.

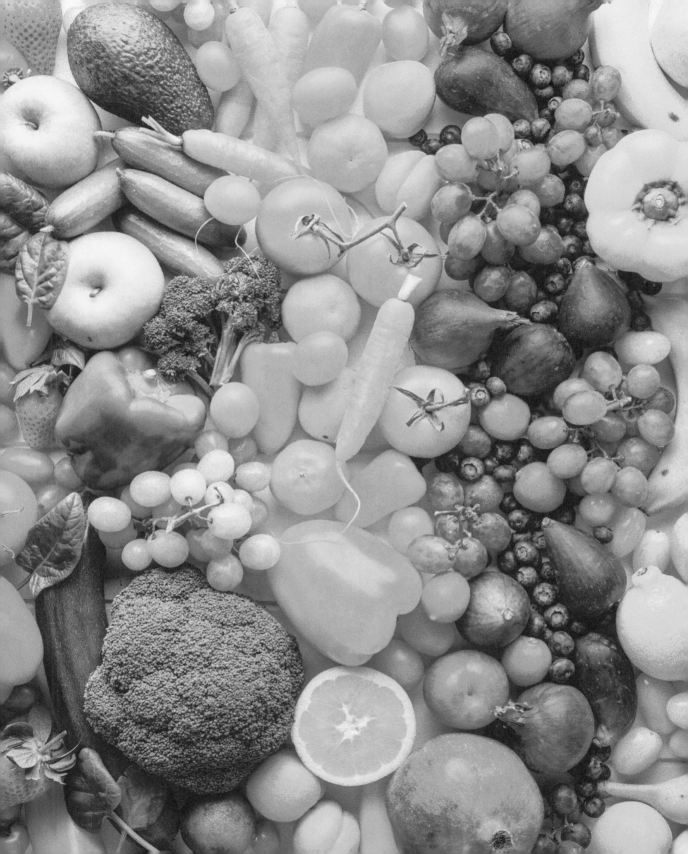

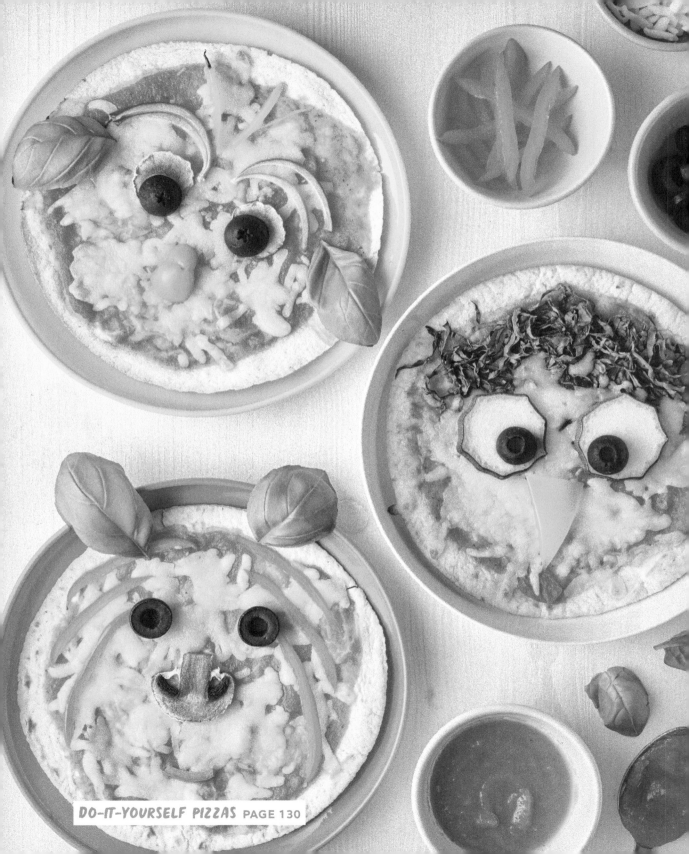

DO-IT-YOURSELF PIZZAS PAGE 130

6

18 MONTHS AND UP

FAMILY MEALS

MOVING FORWARD WITH OPTIMAL NUTRITION

All of a sudden, your beautiful baby is no longer a baby—now, your baby is a child! You have a miniature adult with their own feelings, preferences, and opinions. This tiny one is ready to take their place at the table, right next to you. It's so exciting!

As your little one joins you at the table, they are eating what you eat. Focus on maximizing your own nutrition, as well as the enjoyment of your food choices, and doing so will benefit your child at every level.

LOOKING BEYOND 18 MONTHS

Until your baby was 12 months old, you were stretching and warming up for the big nutrition marathon. From 12 to 18 months, your little one became familiar with your family habits regarding eating and table behavior, while you were starting your marathon. Now you're at the first mile mark and feeling great. Your goal is still way off in the distance, and you'll have a few places where your energy flags, but if you pace yourself you'll be well on the way to the finish line.

Sometimes dinner will be a rainbow of foods presented in a beautiful way, like the Do-It-Yourself Tacos (page 132). Other times, it will be a meal like Home-Cooked Fish Sticks (page 111) that you previously made and froze, but now have defrosted and baked, and you're serving them with cooked frozen mixed veggies. Good nutrition—and good parenting in general—isn't made or broken with a single meal, a single day, or even a single week. It's the culmination of years of adventurous food exposure, joyful meals, and happy togetherness.

IMPORTANT NUTRIENTS

While it's common to continue breastfeeding, during this time, your child's food will meet all their nutritional needs. Throughout childhood, there is a heavy focus on calcium and iron. If your child is drinking cow's milk or consuming fortified non-dairy alternatives, they will likely meet their calcium needs. Iron often comes from meat, but it can also be found in significant amounts in leafy greens, beans, nuts, and seeds. Cooking with a cast-iron pan is also an easy way to increase the iron content in your food.

To make a meal more nutritious, I always like to say, "When in doubt, add a veggie!" Vegetables are nutritious, but they are also colorful and delicious. By seeing each meal as an opportunity to add a plant, you'll maximize your child's nutrition, as well as their exposure to a beautiful plate of food.

Nutrition is full of nuance. When we classify foods as good or bad, that doesn't leave room for nuance. For example, a chocolate chip cookie doesn't yield the nutrition the body needs in the same way that a plate of roasted broccoli will. But does that make a cookie bad? What if that cookie is made by you and your Little Chef together, enjoying laughter and floured noses? What if it's a cookie shared after a difficult day or as part of a birthday or holiday celebration?

When we consider good health, we must include all forms of health: physical, of course, but also emotional, mental, and spiritual health. To that end, choose your food carefully. Put thought into it, but not so much thought that it takes over your days. Once you have chosen the food for a particular meal, enjoy it. Teach your child to season the food with laughter and maybe sesame seeds, not guilt and shame. This will be one of the best lessons you can pass on to your little one.

TYPICAL MEALS AND SCHEDULE

Even as your child begins to naturally condense their nap schedule, routine will continue to be important. Some children will be forgiving if there is a lapse in routine, while others will demand to stay on schedule. You know your child best and can choose what is in their (and your) best interest.

Sample Meal Schedule

6:00 A.M.	Wake up
6:30 A.M.	Breakfast; include 2–3 ounces (¼–⅓ cup) whole milk or non-dairy alternative
9:15 A.M.	Snack 1; include 2–3 ounces (¼–⅓ cup) whole milk or non-dairy alternative
11:30 A.M.	Lunch; include 2–3 ounces (¼–⅓ cup) whole milk or non-dairy alternative
12:00 P.M.	Nap (1½ to 2 hours or more)
2:30 P.M.	Snack 2; include 2–3 ounces (¼–⅓ cup) whole milk or non-dairy alternative
5:00 P.M.	Dinner; include 2–3 ounces (¼–⅓ cup) whole milk or non-dairy alternative
6:00 P.M.	Bedtime

COMMON CHALLENGES

Here are some common challenges that you might face at the 18-month mark.

MY CHILD HAS CHOSEN TO BE A VEGETARIAN!

While we as adults can enjoy a variety of textures, all in a single meal, your little one is just learning. It's like taking the stairs two steps at a time versus slowly crawling up one at a time. Meat often feels dry to little kids. Sometimes you can work around this by providing wetter meats, such as meatballs (like Yaffi's Classic Slow Cooker Meatballs, page 86, or Slow Cooker Chicken Korma, page 137), and similar saucy entrées. Sometimes your child will just opt out. This is when serving a variety comes into play: if you serve grilled chicken breast, rice, and green beans, and your child chooses to eat only the rice and veggies, they will be fine. Even if they choose only the rice, they will be fine. The actual amount of protein children need is much less than we think; a child this age requires only about 13 grams of protein per day. That's equal to one egg and 8 ounces (1 cup) of milk. Continue to offer foods that you enjoy, along with a dish that your child often accepts.

MY CHILD SKIPS DINNER!

This is a very common issue. Kids are super in touch with their internal cues of hunger and fullness. On some days, they grow more; on other days, it's less. On the days when your child experiences rapid growth and development, their appetite will reflect that and they might relish dinner.

I remember making breakfast for my family when my kids were toddlers. They demolished everything I had cooked! On days when your child is growing a bit less, or is coming down with a cold, or recently overcame a big milestone, their appetite may wane. They will arrive at the table having already consumed the nutrition they needed for that day, and their appetite might be less. If there is a two-hour space between dinner and bedtime, offer a boring bedtime snack: apples and cheese, crackers with peanut butter, or fruit and yogurt. Avoid pressuring them to eat in favor of encouraging them to listen to their appetite.

DO-IT-YOURSELF PIZZAS

30 MINUTES OR LESS | **NUT-FREE** | ONE PAN | VEGETARIAN

YIELD: 2 small pizzas **PREP TIME:** 10 minutes **COOK TIME:** 6 minutes

2 (8-inch) pieces of flatbread, such as tortillas, pitas, or lavashes

4 tablespoons low-sodium marinara or pizza sauce

¼ cup shredded mozzarella or ricotta

¼ cup toppings of choice, such as sliced tomato, sliced bell pepper, chopped spinach, sliced garlic, fresh basil, thinly sliced red onion, sliced olives, or sliced mushrooms

At 18 months old, your child is seeking opportunities for independence. The parent's job at the table is to set the boundaries and then to allow the child to grow within those boundaries. This do-it-yourself recipe helps encourage that independence. Including vegetables on the pizza makes it super delicious and beautiful. For little ones, cut the pizza into squares for easier pickup and place a drop cloth under their seat.

1. Preheat the oven to 400°F.

2. Place the flatbreads on a piece of foil or parchment paper set atop a baking sheet. Smear the sauce evenly over the flatbreads, leaving a ½- to 1-inch border around the edge.

3. Sprinkle (or dollop) the cheese over the flatbreads. Evenly distribute the toppings.

4. Bake for 5 to 6 minutes, until the cheese is exactly as melty as you love it.

5. Cool for 3 to 4 minutes, then cut it with a pizza slicer into kid-friendly pieces.

NUTRITION TIP: While pizza gets a bad reputation as a junk food, it contains fat for brain growth and health, calcium for bones, lots of antioxidants in the sauce, fiber in the veggies and flatbread, and most important, the smiles you share as you enjoy a delicious family meal together. Smiles are an underrated health promoter.

DO-IT-YOURSELF QUESADILLAS

30 MINUTES OR LESS | **NUT-FREE** | **ONE PAN** | **VEGETARIAN**

YIELD: 2 quesadillas   **PREP TIME:** 10 minutes   **COOK TIME:** 6 minutes

2 (8-inch) flour
  tortillas
¼ cup shredded
  Monterey
  Jack cheese
¼ cup refried beans
  or mashed low-
  sodium canned
  pinto beans
  (optional)
¼ cup chopped
  vegetables of
  choice, such as
  sliced bell pepper,
  tomato, avocado,
  or corn (optional)
Nonstick
  cooking spray

"That which we call the combination of bread and cheese by any other name would taste as sweet." That's how that line from *Romeo and Juliet* went, right? Let's make that combination Southwest-style for a quesadilla!

1. Lay the tortillas flat on a work surface. Spread the cheese evenly over the tortillas.

2. If you're using beans, spread them over the tortillas as well. If you're going straight for the veggies, distribute those evenly on top of the cheese.

3. Fold one side of each tortilla over the other side for 2 folded tortillas.

4. Preheat an electric griddle to 300°F or preheat a large skillet over medium heat. Coat the cooking surface of either lightly with nonstick cooking spray.

5. Place the tortillas on the griddle or in the skillet and cook for 2 to 3 minutes, until the bottoms begin to brown. Carefully flip them over and cook for another 2 to 3 minutes on the other side.

6. Let cool briefly, then cut each quesadilla in half to serve.

NUTRITION TIP: Beans can be overlooked as a kid-friendly food. They are the perfect size and shape for little fingers just getting their pincer grasp. They are also full of amazing nutrition, including fiber, antioxidants, protein, and folate. If you're mashing some canned beans, give your little one a large bowl and a potato masher and let them go at it!

DO-IT-YOURSELF TACOS

30 MINUTES OR LESS **GLUTEN-FREE** **NUT-FREE** **VEGETARIAN**

YIELD: 8 tacos **PREP TIME:** 5 minutes

1 Hass avocado

1 garlic clove, minced

¼ teaspoon fresh lime juice

8 taco shells

½ cup refried beans or mashed low-sodium canned pinto beans

½ cup frozen corn kernels

1 large tomato, chopped

1 bell pepper, cored, seeded, and chopped

½ cup finely shredded green cabbage

½ cup shredded Monterey Jack cheese

1 lime, cut into wedges

It's Taco Tuesday! Or Maybe it's Friday. No matter what day it is, tacos can always be on the menu. Whether you prefer hard shell, soft tacos, or both—glued together with mashed beans—tacos are the perfect way to get a delicious and nutritious meal from the table to the tummy. By allowing your child to create their own delicious invention, you are establishing appropriate boundaries while also allowing for growth and exploration.

1. Halve the avocado and remove the pit. Scoop the flesh into a small bowl and add the garlic and lime juice, then mash together until combined.

2. Set out the taco shells, beans, corn, tomato, bell pepper, cabbage, and cheese in small bowls or in a divided party platter.

3. Have everyone make their own perfect taco and serve with lime wedges.

ADDITION TIP: You can boost the protein in this veggie-full taco by adding minced leftover chicken or other meat, or by sautéing crumbled firm tofu in a little olive oil and flavoring it with taco seasoning.

LAZY SUSAN DINNER

30 MINUTES OR LESS | **GLUTEN-FREE** | **NUT-FREE**

YIELD: 4 to 6 servings **PREP TIME:** 15 minutes

1 cup sliced cheese,
   shredded cheese,
   or cottage cheese

1 cup cooked
   or canned
   corn kernels

1 cup thawed
   frozen peas

1 cup baby carrots

1 cup cherry
   tomatoes, halved

1 large cucumber,
   sliced

1 cup fresh berries

1 cup cooked
   edamame or
   other bean

Handful of pretzels

2 cups plain full-fat
   Greek yogurt

1 Hass avocado,
   sliced

1 to 2 cups cooked
   rice, quinoa, or
   couscous

1 cup chopped
   cooked chicken,
   tofu, or other
   protein

This dinner is the perfect solution for the night when you need to clean out the refrigerator. You can think of it as "Leftover Night" or "Toddler Tapas Night" if you're feeling saucy. The concept is to put out a bunch of potentially mismatched ingredients and let the family make their own perfect meals, but each ingredient listed is optional!

1. Place all the ingredients on a party platter or in individual small bowls.

2. Encourage family members to serve themselves, making individual combinations.

SUBSTITUTION TIP: Fashion this idea to fit snack time by placing the ingredients in an ice cube tray or muffin tin!

BAKED PASTA CUPS

NUT-FREE **VEGETARIAN**

YIELD: 12 pasta cups **PREP TIME:** 15 minutes **COOK TIME:** 25 minutes

Nonstick cooking
spray
1 tablespoon
minced fresh basil
½ cup (packed)
baby spinach
½ cup chopped
fresh zucchini
½ cup steamed or
roasted broccoli
florets (steamed
or roasted)
8 ounces ziti, rotini,
or macaroni
1 tablespoon
olive oil
1 (16-ounce) jar
low-sodium
marinara or
other sauce
½ cup ricotta
1½ cups shredded
mozzarella

Kids love to help in the kitchen, but at this age there must be some immediate gratification. They won't understand why baking and cooling takes time. This recipe bridges the gap between the fun and the food. Try this early in the afternoon so there is time to develop an appetite after the activity. Why? Because although this game doesn't require the child to take bites, that's always when it happens—when there is no pressure to eat.

1. Preheat the oven to 350°F. Coat a 12-cup muffin tin with cooking spray.

2. Set out bowls with the basil, spinach, zucchini, and broccoli. If you feel comfortable, guide your Little Chef to chop the vegetables a bit more with a toddler-safe knife. (This could be a messy endeavor.)

3. Cook the pasta according to package directions, about 10 minutes, then strain and place in a large bowl. Toss with the olive oil to keep the pasta from sticking.

4. Add the marinara to the pasta and stir in the ricotta. Mix well.

5. Divide the pasta among the muffin cups, filling the cups about three-quarters full. Allow your child to add some chopped vegetables to each cup. Save any leftover veggies.

6. Top each pasta cup with mozzarella cheese and bake for 12 to 15 minutes, until the cheese is melted and the pasta begins to brown at the edges.

7. While the pasta bakes, give your little one a plain paper plate. Sit down with them and create faces on the plate with leftover veggies. Can you make a smile? A surprised face? Can you make a heart or a rainbow?

COOKING TIP: Cooking with kids isn't just about having fun. The confidence a child experiences when they see their own creation set on a plate in front of them is worth the mess. Kids thrive on appropriate responsibility, and you can start this from a very early age!

MUSHROOM BURGERS

30 MINUTES OR LESS **DAIRY-FREE** **GLUTEN-FREE** **NUT-FREE** **ONE PAN**

YIELD: 10 burgers **PREP TIME:** 10 minutes **COOK TIME:** 8 minutes

8 ounces fresh
   mushrooms,
   chopped
1 medium onion,
   chopped
4 garlic cloves,
   minced
1 pound ground beef
1 pound ground
   turkey
3 large eggs
½ cup gluten-free
   old-fashioned
   rolled oats
½ teaspoon
   freshly ground
   black pepper
1 teaspoon
   sweet paprika
1 teaspoon
   onion powder
Nonstick cooking
   spray

Fresh mushrooms in a burger mix have a subtle and savory flavor and a light texture that lends itself so well to a satisfying meal. These burgers are also freezer-friendly; after mixing and forming, seal them in a freezer-safe container and freeze for up to 3 months. These burgers are best served with buns and all the fixings.

1. Combine the mushrooms, onion, and garlic in a food processor until finely chopped.

2. In a large bowl, combine the mushroom mixture with the beef, turkey, eggs, oats, pepper, paprika, and onion powder.

3. Line a baking sheet with parchment paper or wax paper.

4. Using a ⅓-cup measure, scoop up portions of the mixture and form it into balls. Press each ball into a patty shape about ½ inch thick and place on the baking sheet. You should have about 10 burgers.

5. Preheat an electric grill to hot or place a large skillet over medium heat and lightly coat the surface of either with cooking spray. Add the patties and cook until lightly browned, flipping once. They should reach an internal temperature of 165°F, 3 to 4 minutes on each side.

NUTRITION TIP: Mushrooms are full of antioxidants and other vitamins, and can produce vitamin D after being exposed to UV light. Vitamin D isn't found in many foods, and not all mushrooms are a good source of it. Check at your local grocery store to see if they carry the UV-exposed mushrooms, which would be high in vitamin D.

SLOW COOKER CHICKEN KORMA

DAIRY-FREE **GLUTEN-FREE** **NUT-FREE**

YIELD: 6 to 8 servings **PREP TIME:** 20 minutes **COOK TIME:** 4 to 5 hours, unattended

1 tablespoon
ground coriander

1 tablespoon
ground cumin

½ teaspoon ground
turmeric

1 teaspoon
chili powder

1 teaspoon
sweet paprika

½ teaspoon ground
cinnamon

1 teaspoon
kosher salt

2 tablespoons
olive oil

2 medium onions,
diced

1 teaspoon dark or
light brown sugar

2 garlic cloves,
minced

2 teaspoons minced
fresh ginger

1 (13.5-ounce)
can full-fat
coconut milk

2 pounds skinless,
boneless
chicken thighs

Korma is a type of curry, a dish popular in India, traditionally served over rice. This curry is warm and comforting on a cold day. Including these flavors in your child's regular rotation will help ensure a wide variety of accepted tastes and textures.

1. Combine the coriander, cumin, turmeric, chili powder, paprika, cinnamon, and salt in a small bowl.

2. Heat the olive oil in a medium skillet over medium heat. Add the onions and brown sugar and sauté for 2 to 3 minutes, until golden.

3. Add the garlic and ginger and cook for 1 minute more. Then add the spice mixture and cook for 2 minutes, just until spices are toasted and become fragrant.

4. Place the skillet mixture in a blender or food processor and add the coconut milk; blend until smooth.

5. Place the chicken in the slow cooker, pour in the sauce, and cook on low for 4 to 5 hours, until the internal temperature of the chicken is 165°F.

NUTRITION TIP: Vibrant seasonings like turmeric, paprika, and garlic have immense nutritional value. They are known to be anti-inflammatory agents, supporting the immune system and promoting overall health.

ADDITION TIP: If you'd like, add ¼ cup raisins to the slow cooker at step 5.

EGG ROLL-UP BITES

30 MINUTES OR LESS **NUT-FREE** **ONE PAN** **VEGETARIAN**

YIELD: 1 tortilla roll PREP TIME: 5 minutes COOK TIME: 5 to 6 minutes

1 teaspoon unsalted butter or olive oil

½ cup chopped fresh spinach

2 large eggs, lightly beaten

1 tablespoon crumbled feta

1 (10-inch) flour tortilla

This snack concept became popular with chef Nadiya Hussain because of its ease, nutrition, and delicious taste. When you roll this up, listen closely. That's the sound of delicious. Here is my take on this new classic. This recipe makes only one roll-up, but you can easily multiply the ingredients to make several rolls for a family meal.

1. In a medium skillet, melt the butter over medium heat. Add the spinach and sauté until wilted, about 2 minutes.

2. Add the eggs and cook until nearly set. The center will still be a bit jiggly. Sprinkle the feta over the eggs.

3. Lay the tortilla on top of the eggs and press it down into the egg mixture. Using a spatula, flip the whole thing over so the tortilla is on the bottom and the eggs are on top.

4. Cook for 2 to 3 minutes more, or until the bottom of the tortilla begins to brown.

5. Slide the tortilla onto a clean, flat surface. Roll it up, listening carefully for that delicious crackling sound.

6. Using a sharp knife, cut the roll into 4 pieces, sushi-style.

SUBSTITUTION TIP: Experiment with different veggie combinations. You can add things like mushroom and sun-dried tomatoes, asparagus and dill Havarti, or whatever you think sounds delicious!

SLOW COOKER SIMPLE CHICKEN

DAIRY-FREE GLUTEN-FREE NUT-FREE

YIELD: 4 or 5 servings **PREP TIME:** 5 minutes **COOK TIME:** 4 to 6 hours, unattended

1 cup fresh
   orange juice
1 (3½-pound)
   chicken, cut into
   8 pieces
½ teaspoon
   garlic powder
½ teaspoon
   onion powder

This is a "I-have-no-energy-to-cook" dinner. It's also the ultimate chameleon dish—its leftovers can reappear in many different forms, always new and always delicious. Use those leftovers in soup, in a green salad, with rice and veggies, as stir-fry, or as chicken salad. Ease and versatility are the names of this game.

1. Pour the orange juice into the slow cooker.

2. Add the chicken and sprinkle with the garlic and onion powders.

3. Close the cooker and slow-cook on low for 6 hours or on high for 4 hours. The chicken is done when the internal temperature is 165°F.

SUBSTITUTION TIP: Many kids at this age choose to be vegetarian. It's all about the texture. Substituting a slow cooker recipe like this gives chicken a juicy texture that everyone will love.

STUFF-YOUR-OWN SWEET POTATOES

GLUTEN-FREE NUT-FREE VEGETARIAN

YIELD: 4 potatoes **PREP TIME:** 10 minutes **COOK TIME:** 50 minutes

4 medium sweet
   potatoes,
   scrubbed clean
1½ tablespoons
   olive oil
½ medium onion,
   finely diced
1 garlic clove, diced
½ teaspoon ground
   black pepper
¼ teaspoon
   ground cumin
¼ teaspoon
   chili powder
½ teaspoon
   kosher salt
1 (15-ounce) can
   low-sodium black
   beans, drained
   and rinsed
1 Hass avocado,
   cubed
½ cup plain full-fat
   Greek yogurt,
   sour cream,
   or non-dairy
   alternative

Sweet potatoes have beautiful color, creamy texture, and sweet and earthy flavor. This is my favorite way to serve them—plain baked, ready for stuffing.

1. Preheat the oven to 425°F. Line a baking sheet with parchment paper or aluminum foil.

2. Prick each sweet potato 5 to 6 times with a fork and lay on the baking sheet. Bake for 45 to 50 minutes, until a fork inserts easily.

3. Let cool for 10 minutes, then split the sweet potatoes open.

4. While the potatoes are cooling, heat the olive oil in a medium skillet. Add the onion and garlic, and cook for 3 to 4 minutes, until the onion begins to soften.

5. Add the pepper, cumin, chili powder, and salt, and cook for 2 to 3 minutes, until just fragrant.

6. Add the beans and cook until heated through.

7. Split open the sweet potatoes and arrange them on a platter. Place the filling in a separate bowl so family members can spoon as much filling into their potatoes as desired, mixing it with the sweet potato pulp. Serve with the avocado and yogurt.

SUBSTITUTION TIP: Other options for delicious sweet potato stuffings include Elote (page 116), Yaffi's Slow Cooker Lentil Stew (page 146), crumbled Very Veggie Patties (page 84), Baked Salmon Croquettes (page 90), Popcorn Roasted Cauliflower (page 93), Broccoli and Cheddar Quinoa Cups (page 110), and Baked Salmon with Veggies (page 149)!

EGGPLANT PARMESAN MUFFINS

NUT-FREE VEGETARIAN

YIELD: 12 muffins **PREP TIME:** 20 minutes **COOK TIME:** 35 minutes

Nonstick cooking
  spray
1 cup panko
  bread crumbs
2 teaspoons Italian
  seasoning
½ teaspoon
  kosher salt
1 long and narrow
  eggplant, trimmed
1 large egg
1 tablespoon water
1½ cups low-sodium
  marinara sauce
1½ cups shredded
  mozzarella
¾ cup freshly
  grated or shaved
  Parmesan cheese
¾ cup chopped
  fresh basil
  leaves, chopped

These muffin-size bites are a wonderful introduction to cooking with your Little Chef. And they make a great lunch or dinner at home or on the go. When choosing an eggplant, look for one that is smooth, shiny, uniform in color, and heavy for its size. Lightly press a finger against the skin; if it leaves an imprint, the eggplant is asking to be taken home and enjoyed.

1. Preheat the oven to 400°F. Coat a 12-cup muffin tin with cooking spray and line a baking sheet with parchment paper.

2. Spread the bread crumbs evenly over the baking sheet and bake for 4 minutes, stir, then bake for another 2 to 3 minutes, until golden. Place the crumbs in a wide shallow bowl and add the Italian seasoning and salt. Reduce the oven temperature to 350°F and retain the lined baking sheet.

3. Slice the eggplant crosswise into 36 rounds about ¼ inch thick. Using an inverted cup as a guide, trim the slices to equal the diameter of the muffin cups in the tin.

4. In another shallow bowl, whisk the egg with the water.

5. Dip each eggplant round in the egg mixture to coat, then press it into the bread crumbs. Place the slices on the baking sheet.

CONTINUED >

EGGPLANT PARMESAN MUFFINS CONTINUED

6. Into each muffin cup place 1 eggplant round, then add 1 tablespoon of the sauce, 1 tablespoon of the Parmesan, and a sprinkling of fresh basil. Add another layer of eggplant, 1 tablespoon sauce, and 1 tablespoon mozzarella, and finally another eggplant slice and a sprinkling of mozzarella.

7. Cover the muffin tin loosely with aluminum foil and bake for 25 minutes.

8. Remove the foil and bake 5 minutes more, until the tops are golden brown.

NUTRITION TIP: Eggplant is also called aubergine or brinjal in other countries and is botanically a berry. Eggplants are a great source of antioxidants, particularly a type of anthocyanin called nasunin, which is a free-radical scavenger. It protects cells against damage, specifically protecting the brain from cell damage. It is mainly found in the eggplant peel!

DAD'S PEANUT CHICKEN NOODLES

30 MINUTES OR LESS | **DAIRY-FREE**

YIELD: 6 to 8 servings **PREP TIME:** 5 minutes **COOK TIME:** 15 minutes

1 (1-pound) box spaghetti

½ cup creamy natural peanut butter

¼ teaspoon kosher salt

1½ cups chopped cooked chicken

My father is a great cook, but he never writes down his recipes. He made a delicious peanut chicken noodle dish once, but has never been able to re-create it. Here, I give you my closest approximation of his simple but ambrosial invention.

1. Cook the pasta according to package instructions until al dente, about 10 minutes. Drain and set aside. Reserve the cooking water.

2. In a blender or food processor, combine the peanut butter, ½ cup reserved cooking water, and the salt. Blend until smooth.

3. Pour the sauce into a large saucepan, add the pasta and chicken, and heat over moderate heat, stirring to blend well, 5 to 10 minutes.

MEAL TIP: Serve this dish with a brightly colored vegetable, such as roasted broccoli, or a plate of crunchy fresh vegetables.

SUBSTITUTION TIP: You can substitute roasted tofu (see page 87) for the chicken to make this vegetarian.

TRADITIONAL SHAKSHUKA

DAIRY-FREE GLUTEN-FREE NUT-FREE ONE PAN VEGETARIAN

YIELD: 6 servings **PREP TIME:** 10 minutes **COOK TIME:** about 25 minutes

2 tablespoons olive oil

1 large onion, chopped

1 large red bell pepper, cored, seeded, and chopped

¼ teaspoon kosher salt

2 to 3 garlic cloves, thinly sliced or minced

1 teaspoon sweet paprika

½ teaspoon ground cumin

6 vine-ripened tomatoes, chopped, or 1 (28-ounce) can fire-roasted tomatoes

½ cup low-sodium tomato sauce

6 large eggs

Shakshuka may be a food trend right now, but it's been a staple in the Middle East and North Africa for a long time. Top this with some crumbled feta and serve it with toast for a complete meal. Need a shortcut? Many stores now sell a "shakshuka starter," leaving you only with the task of adding the eggs.

1. Heat the oil in a large skillet over medium heat just until it shimmers. Add the onion, bell pepper, salt, and garlic. Cook for 4 to 6 minutes, stirring continuously, until the vegetables are soft.

2. Add the paprika and cumin. Cook for 2 minutes more, until fragrant.

3. Pour in the tomatoes and tomato sauce. (If using canned tomatoes, include the juices.) Stir to blend well, then reduce the heat to a simmer and cook for 5 minutes.

4. Using the back of a spoon, create a well. Crack the eggs, one at a time, directly into the well. (Alternatively, crack the eggs individually into a small measuring cup, then pour the egg into the well.)

5. Cover the skillet loosely with aluminum foil, and cook until desired consistency, 10 minutes for runny yolks, 15 minutes for hardened yolks, or anywhere in between.

SUBSTITUTION TIP: Be sure to use a well-seasoned cast-iron skillet; a new or under-seasoned pan will result in a sticky mess.

POTATO BROCCOLI SOUP

`DAIRY-FREE` `GLUTEN-FREE` `NUT-FREE`

YIELD: 4 to 6 servings **PREP TIME:** 5 minutes, plus 10 minutes to cool
COOK TIME: 25 minutes

1 medium stalk of
    broccoli
2 tablespoons
    olive oil
½ medium
    onion, chopped
1 garlic clove,
    minced
4 cups no- or low-
    sodium chicken or
    vegetable broth
1 large russet
    potato, peeled
    and chopped
Kosher salt and
    freshly ground
    black pepper

The broccoli in this soup lends a bright and cheerful look, while the potatoes make it a cozy hug in a bowl. For color and texture, serve this alongside a plate of crunchy veggies.

1. Cut the florets from the broccoli, then peel the stem and chop it. Cut the floret into small pieces.

2. Heat the oil in a medium saucepan over medium heat. Add the onion and garlic, and cook for 3 to 4 minutes, until the onion begins to soften.

3. Pour in the broth and bring to a boil. Add the broccoli stem and the potato to the pan, reduce the heat to a simmer, and cook for 15 minutes, until the potato is tender.

4. Allow to cool for 10 minutes, then transfer to a blender or use an immersion blender to puree until smooth.

5. Taste and add salt and pepper as needed.

6. Add the broccoli floret and cook until just tender, about 5 minutes.

NUTRITION TIP: I was once told that if you were stranded on a deserted island, broccoli could meet all your nutritional needs. I don't know how true that is, but broccoli is certainly one of my favorite vegetables. It is not only full of nutrition but is also a beautiful color and offers different texture exposures.

YAFFI'S SLOW COOKER LENTIL STEW

DAIRY-FREE **GLUTEN-FREE** **NUT-FREE** **VEGAN**

YIELD: 6 servings **PREP TIME:** 5 minutes **COOK TIME:** 4 hours, unattended

4 cups- or low-
  sodium vegetable
  or chicken broth
1 cup red lentils
1 medium white
  potato, peeled
  and cubed
1 sweet potato,
  peeled and cubed
2 medium
  carrots, sliced
1 celery stalk, sliced
¼ teaspoon
  freshly ground
  black pepper
¼ teaspoon
  ground cumin
¼ teaspoon
  sweet paprika
¼ teaspoon ground
  turmeric
Kosher salt
1 lemon, cut
  into wedges
2 cups (packed)
  chopped
  fresh spinach

I was introduced to lentil stew while working at an Israeli restaurant that employed a Tunisian chef. He taught me that lentils need lemon, and that a thick lentil stew always pairs well with warm pita and creamy hummus. Lentils are a staple in many places around the world, but I enjoy them most as a delicious stew on a cold day.

1. Place the broth, lentils, white and sweet potatoes, carrots, celery, pepper, cumin, paprika, turmeric, and salt to taste in the slow cooker. Cover and cook on low for 4 hours.

2. To serve, divide the stew evenly among bowls and top with a handful of spinach and a squeeze of lemon.

MEAL TIP: This dish contains all the nutrients you'll need for a satisfying meal, but serving the stew with garlic toast or pitas and hummus really takes it into favorite-dinner territory.

MAKE-AHEAD TIP: Leftovers can be stored in an airtight container in the refrigerator for up to 3 days or in the freezer for up to 6 months.

ZUCCHINI PIRATE SHIPS

GLUTEN-FREE | NUT-FREE | ONE PAN | VEGETARIAN

YIELD: 6 servings PREP TIME: 10 minutes COOK TIME: 25 minutes

3 medium zucchini, halved lengthwise

Nonstick cooking spray

1 cup cooked brown rice

1 cup cooked brown lentils

½ cup cherry tomatoes, halved

½ small red onion, chopped

3 tablespoons red wine vinegar

2 tablespoons olive oil

1 tablespoon fresh lemon juice

1 teaspoon dried oregano

2 garlic cloves, minced

¼ teaspoon freshly ground black pepper

¼ teaspoon kosher salt

½ cup tzatziki (optional)

Who doesn't like dinner served in a boat? Maybe it's a pirate ship with a celery cannon. Or maybe it's a spaceship with little mushroom aliens. Don't be afraid to play with your food—really! Making fun out of dinner can help a hesitant eater feel confident.

1. Preheat the oven to 400°F.

2. Scoop out the center of each zucchini half to create a boat. Coat a 9-by-13-inch glass baking dish with cooking spray, then arrange the zucchini boats in the dish.

3. In a large bowl, combine the rice, lentils, tomatoes, onion, vinegar, olive oil, lemon juice, oregano, garlic, pepper, and salt.

4. Evenly scoop the stuffing mixture into the zucchini boats, mounding it up and smoothing the tops.

5. Bake, uncovered, for 20 to 25 minutes, or until the zucchini are tender when poked with a fork. Remove from the oven and top with tzatziki, if desired.

NUTRITION TIP: Zucchini often acts as a stand-in for something else, but in this recipe it takes on a main role—as it should. Zucchini, like eggplant, is botanically a fruit! It is surprisingly high in vitamin C, which helps support immunity, and vitamin B_6, which helps support mood and brain health.

TANTE SUZY'S CHICKEN NOODLE SOUP

DAIRY-FREE **NUT-FREE**

YIELD: 6 to 8 servings **PREP TIME:** 15 minutes, plus 10 minutes to cool
COOK TIME: about 3 hours

1 (1-pound)
   package thin
   egg noodles
2 tablespoons
   olive oil
1 large onion
1 (3½-pound)
   chicken, cut into
   8 pieces
2 small parsnips,
   peeled and
   chopped
1 medium leek,
   trimmed and
   chopped
3 to 5 medium
   carrots, chopped
3 to 5 celery
   stalks, chopped
Generous handful
   of fresh parsley,
   chopped
3 tablespoons
   chopped fresh dill
2 teaspoons kosher
   salt, or more
   as needed

Suzy took care of me when my twins were born. During that difficult time, she was a friend, confidante, and bearer of all things nurturing. This is her delicious chicken soup.

1. Cook the noodles according to the package directions until al dente, about 8 minutes. Drain and place in a bowl. Toss with the olive oil.

2. Remove the outer papery peel from the onion, leaving some of the yellow skin.

3. Put the chicken and onion into a large stockpot, add enough water to cover the chicken, cover the pot, and slowly boil, covered, for 1 hour.

4. Stir in the parsnips, leek, carrots, celery, parsley, dill, and salt. Simmer, covered, for 2 to 3 hours.

5. Turn off the heat. Using tongs, remove the chicken and let it cool in the refrigerator. When cool enough to handle, remove the meat from the bones and discard, along with the skin. If desired, skim any fat from the top of the broth.

6. Place the chicken meat back in the stockpot with the broth and add the noodles. Bring to a simmer over low heat to warm through before serving.

NUTRITION TIP: Chicken soup has been called "Jewish Penicillin" because of its tryptophan and other micronutrients. Research backs it up this ancient knowledge!

BAKED SALMON WITH VEGGIES

`DAIRY-FREE` `GLUTEN-FREE` `NUT-FREE` `ONE PAN`

YIELD: 4 servings **PREP TIME:** 10 minutes **COOK TIME:** 1 hour

Nonstick cooking spray (optional)

2 pounds small red or yellow potatoes, quartered

½ teaspoon kosher salt, divided

½ teaspoon freshly ground black pepper, divided

4 garlic cloves, minced, divided

3 tablespoons olive oil

¼ cup fresh lemon juice

4 (6-ounce) wild-caught salmon fillets

6 medium Brussels sprouts, trimmed and cut into ¼-inch slices

1 small red bell pepper, cored, seeded, and cut into ¼-inch-thick strips

I never liked salmon when I was growing up. That would come as a shock to anyone who knows me now. Salmon is cooked to an internal temperature of 145°F—any less, and it's still raw, and any more, and it's dry. But at 145°F, it's flaky, buttery, and delicious.

1. Preheat the oven to 400°F. Line a half-sheet pan with parchment paper or use aluminum foil and coat it with cooking spray.

2. Lay the potatoes in the pan in a single layer. Season with ¼ teaspoon each of salt and black pepper, and sprinkle with 2 of the garlic cloves.

3. Bake for 25 minutes, until the potatoes can be pierced easily with a fork.

4. Meanwhile, in a small bowl, combine the olive oil, the remaining 2 garlic cloves, the lemon juice, and the remaining ¼ teaspoon each of salt and black pepper.

5. In a medium bowl, toss the Brussels sprouts and red bell pepper with 3 tablespoons of dressing.

CONTINUED >

BAKED SALMON WITH VEGGIES CONTINUED

6. Remove the sheet pan from the oven and shift the potatoes to the sides. Spread the Brussels sprouts and bell pepper slices among the potatoes.

7. Place the salmon fillets skin side down in the middle of the pan. Brush the tops of the salmon with the remaining dressing and bake for 15 to 18 minutes, until the salmon measures 145°F and the Brussels sprouts are tender and crisped.

NUTRITION TIP: Salmon is a great source of DHA, so it's important for developing brains. The Dietary Guidelines for Americans recommends at least 8 ounces of a low-mercury fish per week. Salmon is a great addition to your weekly rotation.

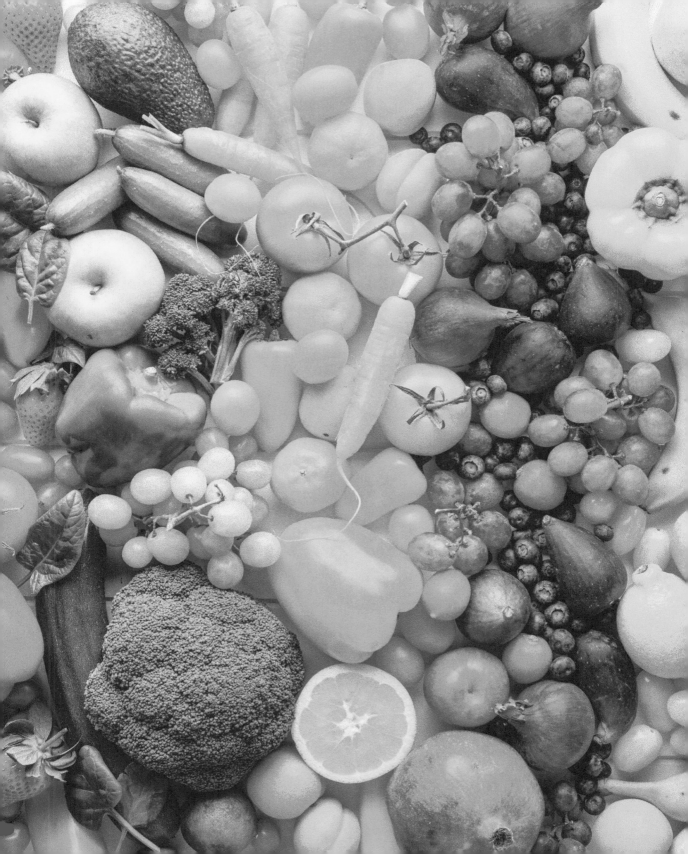

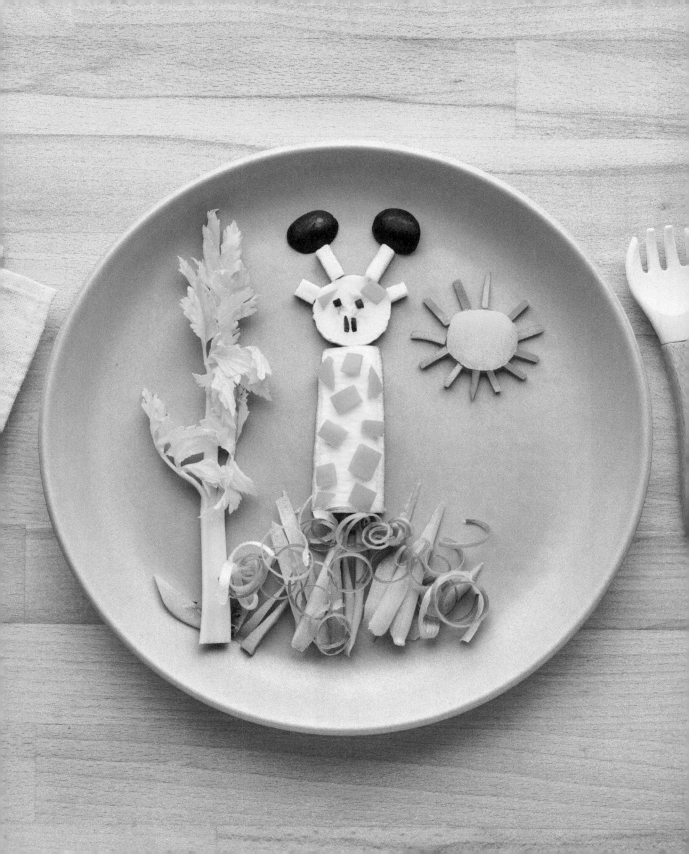

MEASUREMENT CONVERSIONS

VOLUME EQUIVALENTS (LIQUID)

US STANDARD	US STANDARD (OUNCES)	METRIC (APPROXIMATE)
2 tablespoons	1 fl. oz.	30 mL
¼ cup	2 fl. oz.	60 mL
½ cup	4 fl. oz.	120 mL
1 cup	8 fl. oz.	240 mL
1 ½ cups	12 fl. oz.	355 mL
2 cups or 1 pint	16 fl. oz.	475 mL
4 cups or 1 quart	32 fl. oz.	1 L
1 gallon	128 fl. oz.	4 L

OVEN TEMPERATURES

FAHRENHEIT	CELSIUS (APPROXIMATE)
250°F	120°C
300°F	150°C
325°F	165°C
350°F	180°C
375°F	190°C
400°F	200°C
425°F	220°C
450°F	230°C

VOLUME EQUIVALENTS (DRY)

US STANDARD	METRIC (APPROXIMATE)
⅛ teaspoon	0.5 mL
¼ teaspoon	1 mL
½ teaspoon	2 mL
¾ teaspoon	4 mL
1 teaspoon	5 mL
1 tablespoon	15 mL
¼ cup	59 mL
⅓ cup	79 mL
½ cup	118 mL
⅔ cup	156 mL
¾ cup	177 mL
1 cup	235 mL
2 cups or 1 pint	475 mL
3 cups	700 mL
4 cups or 1 quart	1 L

WEIGHT EQUIVALENTS

US STANDARD	METRIC (APPROXIMATE)
½ ounce	15 g
1 ounce	30 g
2 ounces	60 g
4 ounces	115 g
8 ounces	225 g
12 ounces	340 g
16 ounces or 1 pound	455 g

RESOURCES

NUTRITION FOR RAISING CHILDREN

NAPTIMENUTRITION.COM: Free and relevant information on parenting, children, and nutrition. Use the search tab or playlists to explore topics including gluten, fat, pumping, how to read growth charts, and so much more!

EXPERIENCEDELICIOUSNOW.COM: See Arielle Dani Lebovitz's growing collection of food-based art books and freebies.

FOOD INTRODUCTION

Lvova, Yaffi, RDN. *Stage-by-Stage Baby Food Cookbook: 100+ Purees and Baby-Led Feeding Recipe for a Healthy Start* (Emeryville, CA: Rockridge Press, 2020).

FEEDINGLITTLES.COM: Feeding Littles has wonderful online courses on both baby-led weaning and toddler feeding. Check https://babybloomnutrition.com /additional-support for sales or discount codes.

CHILD NUTRITION

ELLYNSATTERINSTITUTE.ORG: Ellyn Satter, MS, RD, MSSW, developed the Division of Responsibility in her feeding model. Her site is a valuable resource for further information on guiding your child toward a healthy relationship with food and body.

FEEDINGBYTES.COM: Natalia Stasenko, RD and feeding expert, provides up-to-date, convenient resources on her website and social media outlets.

YOURFEEDINGTEAM.COM: Natalia Stasenko, Jo Cormack, and Simone Emery have teamed up to provide guidance for parents overcoming the obstacles of picky eating.

THEFEEDINGDOCTOR.COM: Katja Rowell, MD, provides books, blogs, and other free resources on child nutrition, extreme picky eating, food preoccupation, and much more.

HEALTHYCHILDREN.ORG: The American Academy of Pediatrics parenting website provides reliable health information about children and parenting.

Lvova, Yaffi, RDN. *Fun with Food Toddler Cookbook: Activities and Recipes to Play and Eat* (Emeryville, CA: Rockridge Press, 2021).

Lvova, Yaffi, RDN. *Beyond a Bite: Activities for a Mindful Mealtime* (self-pub, 2020).

NUTRITION FOR THE SENSORY SENSITIVE CHILD

NAUREENHUNANI.COM: Information and advice from Naureen Hunani, RD.

ROOTSPEDIATRICTHERAPY.COM: Information from Hana Eichele, MOT, OTR/L.

Lvova, Yaffi, RDN. *Beyond a Bite Neurodiverse Edition: Joyful Activities for Sensory Food Exploration* (self-pub, 2021).

BABY WEARING

Baby Wearing International is a resource for all things babywearing. They have trained coaches, as well as a lending library. Find the chapter of this organization in your area and regain access to both hands!

BREASTFEEDING

ILCA.ORG: The International Lactation Consultants Association has a search function to help connect you with an international board-certified lactation consultant. Having an advocate during this amazing time can provide important relief.

CRYSTALKARGES.COM/MAMAANDSWEETPEANUTRITION.COM: Find reliable and compassionate advice on breastfeeding and breastfeeding nutrition from these two registered dietitians.

BABY SLEEP

GETQUIETNIGHTS.COM: Tracy Spackman provides gentle sleep coaching information. See her blog for daily schedules with alternative options.

REFERENCES

Adams, Zoe. "25 Interesting Facts About Peas." The Fact Site. July 29, 2020. thefactsite
.com/interesting-pea-facts.

American Academy of Pediatrics. "Responsive Feeding: Set Your Baby Up for Healthy
Growth and Development." Fact sheet. American Academy of Pediatrics, 2019.
ihcw.aap.org/Documents/Early%20Feeding/Responsive%20Feeding/AAP-Respon-
sive-Feeding_Print-Fact-Sheet.pdf.

Anaphylaxis Campaign. "Outgrowing Food Allergy." September 11, 2020. anaphylaxis
.org.uk/knowledgebase/outgrowing-food-allergy.

Bingemann, Theresa. "Practical Peanut Introduction." Newsletter. *American
Academy of Pediatrics*, December 4, 2020. aappublications.org/news/2019/05/28
/practical-peanut-introduction-pediatrics-5-28-19.

Center for Food Safety and Applied Nutrition. "Advice About Eating Fish."
US Food and Drug Administration, August 31, 2020. fda.gov/food/consumers/
advice-about-eating-fish.

Delaware, Judy, and Megan McNamee. "Feeding Littles Favorite Utensils." Feeding
Littles, August 7, 2019. feedinglittles.com/blog/our-favorite-utensils.

———. "Mouth Stuffing and Food Pocketing in Young Children." Feeding Littles, June 26,
2018. feedinglittles.com/blog/mouth-stuffing-and-food-pocketing-in-young-children.

———. "Sweet Berry Constipation Smoothie." Feeding Littles, June 13, 2018. feedinglittles
.com/blog/sweet-berry-constipation-smoothie.

Garlick, P. J. "Protein Requirements of Infants and Children." Nestlé Nutrition Workshop
Series Pediatric Program, 2006. doi:10.1159/000095009.

Healthbeat. "Importance of Potassium." Harvard Health Publishing, 2020. health.harvard
.edu/staying-healthy/the-importance-of-potassium.

HealthyChildren.org. "Discontinuing the Bottle." HealthyChildren.org, 2019.
healthychildren.org/English/ages-stages/baby/feeding-nutrition/Pages
/Discontinuing-the-Bottle.aspx.

Hoecker, Jay L. "How Much Tummy Time Does Your Baby Need?" Mayo Clinic, Mayo Foundation for Medical Education and Research, August 18, 2020. mayoclinic.org /healthy-lifestyle/infant-and-toddler-health/expert-answers/tummy-time/ faq-20057755.

Kaefer, Christine M., and John A Milner. "The Role of Herbs and Spices in Cancer Prevention." *Journal of Nutritional Biochemistry*, June 2008. US National Library of Medicine. ncbi.nlm.nih.gov/pmc/articles/PMC2771684.

Kristy's Cottage. "How to Give Your Baby a Tummy Massage. " Kristy's Cottage, December 15, 2020. kristyscottage.com/tummy-massage-for-baby.

Lvova, Yaffi. *Fun with Food Toddler Cookbook*. Emeryville, CA: Rockridge Press, 2021.

National Health Service. "Iron." *NHS Choices*, 2020. nhs.uk/conditions/vitamins -and-minerals/iron.

National Institutes of Health, " Zinc." Office of Dietary Supplements, US Department of Health and Human Services, July 15, 2020. ods.od.nih.gov/factsheets/Zinc -HealthProfessional.

———National Institutes of Health. "Vitamin D." Office of Dietary Supplements, US Department of Health and Human Services, March 24, 2020. ods.od.nih.gov /factsheets/VitaminD-Consumer.

Olivier, Michelle. "10 Eco-Friendly Feeding Products for Baby (That Are Cute!)." *Baby Foode*, April 19, 2019. babyfoode.com/ blog/10-eco-friendly-feeding-essentials-for-baby.

Rivera, Meseidy. "Everything You Need to Know About Plantains." *The Pioneer Woman*, October 29, 2020. thepioneerwoman.com/food-cooking/recipes/a77725/whats-the -deal-with-plantains.

Spackman, Tracy. "Schedules: Finding the Right One for Your Baby." Get Quiet Nights, 2019. getquietnights.com/schedules-finding-the-right-one-for-your-baby.

Whitney, Alyse. "What's the Difference Between a Sweet Potato and a Yam?" *Bon Appétit*, September 13, 2017. bonappetit.com/story/difference-between-sweet-potato-and-yam.

INDEX

ACKNOWLEDGMENTS

This book was written entirely during the COVID-19 pandemic lockdown of 2020.

I would like to thank the Lev of my life and our wonderful children, Shimon, Benjamin, and Daniel, for joining me in our bunker. Many thanks to our homeschool podlets and to our fearless leader, Shoshi Shachar. Thank you to my parents, Joan and Lenny Kalmenson, for their ongoing support.

I would also like to thank those who helped this book become a reality: Aleesia Gooslin, intern extraordinaire; Laura Apperson; Bracha Kopstick, RD; and everyone else on the Callisto team.

Finally, I would like to thank my sanity. There still remains a shred. I think.

ABOUT THE AUTHOR

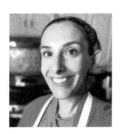

YAFFI LVOVA is a Registered Dietitian Nutritionist and owner of Baby Bloom Nutrition® and Toddler Test Kitchen.™ She holds degrees in both comparative religions and nutrition and dietetics from Arizona State University.

After a difficult journey toward and into motherhood, Yaffi became a mother to twins plus one, and she used her experience and clinical knowledge to shift gears, providing nutrition education to new and expecting parents and helping smooth the transition into parenthood.

In 2015, Yaffi created Toddler Test Kitchen (toddlertestkitchen.net) with immense help from Claudine Wessel, LaKeta Kemp, and Sarah Garone. This unique culinary adventure puts small children in the driver's seat—or at the cutting board as it were—helping bolster self-esteem as they feed their curiosity by creating something delicious!

In 2016, Yaffi went live with a weekly Facebook segment and subsequent podcast, *Nap Time Nutrition* (naptimenutrition.com), covering all topics parenthood and nutrition.

In 2019, Yaffi was brought on board for the update of *Discover Mindful Eating for Kids,* with Megrette Fletcher.

In 2020, Yaffi published *Stage-By-Stage Baby Food Cookbook* and *Beyond a Bite: Activities for a Mindful Mealtime. Beyond a Bite Neurodiverse Edition: Joyful Activities for Sensory Food Exploration* and *Fun with Food Toddler Cookbook: Activities and Recipes to Play and Eat* are planned for publication in 2021.

You can find Yaffi at BabyBloomNutrition.com. On Facebook, she is @BabyBloomNutrition and @ToddlerTestKitchenAZ. On Instagram, you can find her at @toddler.testkitchen. On Twitter she is Yaffi Lvova @BabyBloomNutrit.

CPSIA information can be obtained
at www.ICGtesting.com
Printed in the USA
JSHW030128270421
13897JS00001B/1